Bedtime Stor:

Fall Asleep While Reducing Stress, Worry & Anxiety

by Dan Jones

Connect with Dan Jones:
www.YouTube.com/DanJonesHypnosis

Twitter: @AuthorDanJones

First Edition 2018

Published by Dan Jones

Copyright © Dan Jones 2018

Daniel Jones asserts the moral right to be identified as the author of this work

All rights reserved. No part of this publication may be reproduced, stored in a retrieval system, or transmitted, in any form or by any means, electronic, mechanical, photocopying, recording, or otherwise, without the prior written permission of the publishers or author.

Cover Design by James, GoOnWrite.com

ISBN 978-1724938435

FIRST EDITION

Acknowledgements

This book wouldn't be here if it wasn't for my *Dan Jones Hypnosis* YouTube channel subscribers. As well as thanking Sam Piper and my wife Abbie Jones for their support and help in writing this book, I would also like to thank all of my YouTube subscribers. There isn't enough room to list you all, so here are the 150 subscribers who have contributed most in comments, story ideas and feedback:

AK, Allie L, Amanda Ashton, Amanda Bard, Amber726, Amy, Andrea C, Angela Butler, Ann, Mahnke, Anna Mason, Anna Whetsel Rucker, Anne Kennedy, Anniexhx, Apotofbasil, April M, Askel Sharkowski, B Lebleu, Barking Mad, Becky Badzek, Beth Bachet, Black R05E Tarot, Brandi Dennett, Bug Me, Carly Few, Carole Cochrane, Casey Milano, Cassandra Thompson, Cathy Greenwood, Chanuska Yoha, Charlotte White, Chillin Bro, Cj Seymour, CjLaw, Clare Stephanie, Coleton Humphrey, Crystal Wolfe, D Hanscom, D M, Dana Price, Daphne Hopwood, Derrick

Buxton, Diane Dizayee, Diane Dopp, Dreama Collins, Elfriede Parsons, Elizabeth Anne, Emilia Rigensborg, Emmy See, Empath Soul, Erika L, Evan Wehr, Fabricio Zambon, Flights of Whimzee, Funkynata, Gareth O'Malley, Genesis Whitmore, Genevieve A, Gillian O'Neal, Haley Pemp, Haylee Long, Henry Beach, Holly Fenwick, Honeyydo, IANOYTYK, J B, Jack Morton, Jaimee Elkins, James Lafferty, Jane S, Jay McAvinew, Jennifer Chadwick, Jennifer Richardson, Jennifer Stevenson, Jessica Munro, Jessie Star, Joe Holtz, Joni Brown, Jot1down 1234, Judy, Kandy Celeste Elizabeth Lepe, Kap's Velvet Hammer, Kathleen Cooper, Kay Plumb, Kccustomuph, Kelly Highman, Kveach89, KyahTheAuthor, Leah Jerez, Lee Johnson, Les Kaye, Lifer38, Linda Barclay, Linda Bonine, Lisa O'Keefe, Lisa Warnock, Lisa White-Pagano, LSUchik420, Madam Curious, Magenta Morning, Mana Asj, Margaret Deans, Marissa Boatwright, Mark Morlan, Matti Nightingale, MattsHair, Melanie MacdonalD, Melissa Gibbons, Michael Scofield, Michele Isom, Mirmon, Mizz A, Monday Crawford, Mook A. Burns, MrOscarpolly, Nena Gravil, Niamh Mooney, Nichola Lloyd, Nicole Mackenzie, Noname Foru, Norm Lemans,

Nyla Vox ASMR, Philip Williams, Phyllis Owens, R.E. Daily, Rachel Hlozan, Roberta Maria Atti, Roxanne McIntyre, Ruane Johnson, Seth Rounsavall, Sharon Anderson, Sharon Silljer, Shockvaluecola, Sir Edmund Zeidler, SlamBerry P, Snovakattack1, Spacepadalien, Speak English, Star Lover, StoHelit7, Storm Angel, Strip Down, Sublime, Tabitha Lowney, Tammy W, The Wushu Diamon, Tracy Vieth, Victoria H-B, Wyn Neal, Xaz Shepard, Yvonne Buchanan.

Contents

Introduction	07
Lake of Inner Discovery	25
The Astronaut's Wonder	35
A Lesson in Harmony	42
A Relaxing Break	55
The Sculpture Insight	65
The Student's Dream	75
Connecting with Nature	86
The Couple's 'Frozen in Time' Trip	96
Daddy and Daughter's Fishing Trip	107
Down the Prehistoric Rabbit Hole	118
Falling Asleep in a Rainforest	128
Time Waits for No Man	135
Finding Happiness	149
Finding Wisdom	164
Girl on a Country Walk	174
Legend of the Book of Knowledge	185
Life as an Oak Tree	198
Life on Mars	205
Lost City in the Woods	215
Past-Life Regression	229

Bedtime Stories for Grown-ups

INTRODUCTION

In my early twenties I worked in residential children's homes. One issue we often had was that the children didn't settle well at night. Many of them had experienced abuse and so being in a bedroom and going to sleep caused them anxiety. At bedtime myself and other staff would read the children bedtime stories. It was common that staff would finished reading to the children and would leave their room, but they would still be wide awake and often straight up out of bed running around and being aggressive.

I had been studying hypnosis since I was 14 years old. I didn't know I was autistic at the time, but I did know I struggled with understanding people and hypnosis was the subject that taught me the skills which weren't taught in school that it seemed I was expected to somehow instinctively know. Most nights I would leave a child's room having read a story to them and the other staff would ask what I was doing different, because often the children I read stories to were asleep at the end of the story. I explained that it was how I was reading the stories that was different. I was applying my knowledge of hypnosis to my reading of the stories.

This approach was very successful at helping children settle. After I stopped working in children's homes and started working supporting parents of children with challenging behaviour, I started to teach my storytelling approach to parents. The idea was for them to take any story the child wanted read to them and then read it in a *hypnotic* way. As an example of this hypnotic approach to storytelling I had written a story – *The Rabbit Who Came to Tea* in a parenting book I wrote in 2006 that was written specifically to fit with the hypnotic approach and demonstrate the approach. How I usually did it, was to just read whatever a child wanted read and would read it *hypnotically*. Parents told me that they found this difficult to do in *real-time.* They asked if I could write my own children's stories around the approach so that all the hypnosis and techniques for helping people sleep were contained within the stories, rather than taking a normal story and having to work out how to use the various techniques while reading. So I wrote *Sleepy Bedtime Tales* in 2015 which is a collection of eleven bedtime stories to help children sleep and followed this up with *Relaxing Tales for Children* in 2016 which is another collection of eleven stories. These hypnotic stories for children take about ten minutes to read, which is a suitable length to give time for most children to be asleep by the time the parent finishes reading the story. For adults with sleep problems, generally, the stories need to be longer, 20-30 minutes long is suitable for most adults.

I have always made hypnotic bedtime stories for myself to help me fall asleep. I have difficulty shutting my mind off. I am always thinking of new ideas and inventions, exploring different subjects with curiosity when I should be sleeping. In about 2005 I audio recorded myself a 50-minute story *Adventure of a Prince*. This was the first *bedtime story for grownups* that I had made available for other people to listen to. I had it available on *Myspace* and then *Google Video* and when I joined *YouTube* in 2007 I uploaded it there over six videos (there was a 10-minute video length limit back in those days) and people had to listen the six-part playlist.

I now have over 100 healing hypnotic bedtime stories on my *Dan Jones Hypnosis* YouTube channel (including the twenty stories in this book) which at the time of writing receive over 250,000 views per month. The idea of bedtime stories for grown-ups wasn't always so popular. For the first few years on YouTube I posted a new story every few months, often spending weeks audio recording the story, then creating custom background music and sound effects to match the story and people would comment that bedtime stories are for children, not grownups and say that they didn't understand what I was posting. This isn't uncommon on YouTube, in 2007 I used to post vlogs and videos of me talking about things I had bought, people would comment on asking why would anyone be interested in seeing someone talking to a camera about what they are

Introduction

getting up to and just chatting. Why would anybody be interested in seeing what someone else has bought? This is very common on YouTube now. A few years ago, suddenly the stories I posted became the most popular videos I was posting on my channel. For years, the most popular videos on my channel were my educational videos teaching hypnosis and psychotherapy, my second most popular videos were my self-help and self-hypnosis therapeutic videos, the bedtime stories didn't get very many views.

Over the last few years sleep problems have been on the rise with almost 40% of people in the UK struggling to get enough sleep. Anxiety, worrying and feelings of excessive stress have also been on the increase. These are the main problems behind most people's difficulty sleeping, they have a lot of thoughts, often worrying thoughts, playing on their mind. Due to this they don't feel physiologically relaxed at bedtime due to being stressed and anxious throughout the day. As well as focusing on helping people sleep, these are areas that my bedtime stories cover. The aim is that with time, those using the stories find themselves naturally worrying less, feeling calmer and less stressed, as well as finding themselves drifting off to sleep quicker and easier.

Another problem which listeners of my stories often report causes them sleep problems is pain. Due to the hypnotic nature of the bedtime stories many people find freedom from their pain and find they can sleep even though many of the stories aren't specifically focused on pain management.

This is a collection of twenty *healing hypnotic bedtime stories for grown-ups* from my *Dan Jones Hypnosis* YouTube channel. The average length of the audio for these stories is about 25 minutes per story. Each story contains an introduction and then hypnotic elements designed to help the listener fall asleep. The stories also contain therapeutic elements to address worry, anxiety and managing stress as well as helping with improving sleep and the *Finding Happiness* story also helps with weight loss.

What is Hypnosis?

Many people misunderstand hypnosis. It is a commonly held belief that hypnosis is about suggestion and manipulation and that hypnosis enables some kind of mind control over the person being hypnotised. This couldn't be further from the truth. It is common for people to be less suggestible under hypnosis because hypnosis increases awareness. What this means is that if the hypnotist is trying to manipulate you in some way you are more aware of this than you are when not hypnotised and more likely to refused to follow the manipulation. You aren't unconscious when you are hypnotised and you remember things just as much as you do in everyday life. Hypnosis is just about focusing attention. All a hypnotist is doing is guiding your focus of attention and in the same way that it is easier for someone to park a car when they turn off the radio and ask the passengers to get out of the car and leave so that they can focus all of their attention just on parking, you do better at things when you pay them your full attention. So someone paying all of their attention to quitting smoking will do better at quitting. Someone paying all of their attention to mentally rehearsing being confident when giving a presentation will learn to do better when giving that presentation.

This is all hypnosis does, it focus's attention. There is nothing magical or mystical. This isn't to downplay hypnosis, but to point out the power of focused attention. Hypnosis can't make you do things you don't want to do, you have control over your decisions at all times. All hypnosis does is helps you focus your attention so that you are better able to do that which you are concentrating on.

How do the Stories Work?

The stories all take about 20 to 35 minutes to read when read at a slow comfortable pace with regular pauses to allow the listener to absorb and respond to the ideas presented. This length is generally suitable for most adults to fall asleep to. The introduction to each story is an important hypnotic process, as it establishes how the listener responds to the following story. The introduction presupposes no doubt that the person will fall asleep, the question is how, not if.

As mentioned, one of the main issues people struggling with sleep have, is where their attention is focused. It could be focused on pain, on worrying, on feelings of anxiety or restlessness, or internal mental chatter. For the person to sleep their attention needs to be on just one thing. This thing needs to be calm and not involve any conscious effort or create any conscious stress. One of the first things people often do as they fall asleep is drift into light mental imagery a bit like a daydream. Another thing is that they stop paying attention to their body and their body begins to physiologically relax. So, the stories have to stimulate these areas. They do this by encouraging focus on the sensory components of the presented story and repeatedly directing the listeners attention around aspects of the story so that they aren't focusing on non-story related thoughts and ideas. This process of focusing attention is doing hypnosis. There is no hypnotic induction, it is taking the principles of hypnosis and applying them to encouraging sleep, rather than guiding the listener into hypnosis.

There are other things which deepen inner focus and so encourage sleep. They are using movement – like journeys, travelling and transitions – like walking through a door, or changing scene in some way. This is why the stories often have walking through somewhere, like perhaps a forest, or meadow, or along a beach and why they often have a number of transitions which could be as simple as walking through a door, or from a meadow into woodland. Also to more complex transitions like sitting drinking a drink and finding yourself drifting off into a reverie, or gazing into the sky wondering whether there could be someone out there on another planet, gazing out there wondering whether there is someone out there gazing up into the night sky or finding yourself on another planet gazing out at an alien night sky.

There are various hypnotic techniques used throughout the stories to keep the flow going. You can think of nearly everything given as being built on everything which came before it. This constant building where one thing leads to the next, which leads to the next actually increases absorption in the story, encouraging sleep and the therapeutic work. One of the main techniques used to do this is called linking suggestions. These take a few forms, one is using *and, as, while, during, before, after, when* and other similar connecting words. This is why many sentences start with *and*, which you wouldn't normally have happen in most stories, because the sentence is building on the previous sentence. It is almost like the whole thing is one continuous sentence which just happens to have some full stops and commas interspersed throughout it to give periods of differing lengths of pauses.

Another common linking process is using repetition. I may say something and then say something similar, or even the same thing as the start of the next sentence so that it compounds one on to the other. For example "and then you see a door and as you see that door you decide to walk over to it…" so something has been introduced into the experience and then mentioned again with how it relates to the story.

Another technique used is changing tense or perspective, so I may talk about *they,* or *he, she, her, him* and then at certain points say *you*. I do this when that part is linked to the person experiencing the story or where it is to be linked to them, rather than perhaps just the character of the story. Sometimes this is subtle, but what I find is that it stands out more when reading the stories than it does when experiencing the stories. I may change tense at the same time, so I could say "they walked through the cavern and found an open book, they reached down and picked up the book and started to turn the pages. And as you turn the pages, you notice something strange about this book…" There are also many other techniques being used.

As well as helping people sleep, these stories are designed to help people therapeutically, mainly around tackling anxiety, worry and stress. To do this I utilise the brains innate pattern-matching ability. The brain is an incredible pattern-matching machine. What this means is that it can recognise the underlying pattern regardless of the overlaying content and if those underlying patterns are relevant in the moment then the brain will respond to them. For example, if I walked up to someone in the street and presented patterns for sleep they wouldn't respond to those patterns unless sleep was on their mind, but if the same thing is presented at bedtime when the person wants to sleep they will connect with the sleep patterns.

There are only a limited number of different types of stories that can be written and yet every year millions of new books and films are released which all contain very different content but share similar underlying patterns. So, if someone had a problem where they were trying to look at it to find a solution, but because they are in the problem they struggle to see the solution I can tell a story about someone climbing a mountain and looking out over the view from the top and the person will recognise this pattern in relation to their presenting problem. They will also recognise they need to gain perspective of their problem and will apply this pattern to the problem so that non-consciously they start *viewing* the problem from a new perspective. In reality climbing a mountain would have more patterns than just this. There is the struggle to the top, perhaps a pattern for enjoying the journey and that the journey is as important as the destination, perhaps they get help on their journey, or have rests on the journey. All of these are therapeutic patterns which the brain responds to.

This idea of using patterns in stories to lead to change in the listener isn't new and is something we are all familiar with. For example, most people probably know the story of the ugly duckling and through all of human history, stories have been told containing patterns for how to live life, learn lessons and deal with challenges. Some patterns are obvious, others are less so because we generally don't spend our time thinking about our challenges and working out the patterns of them and then taking that pattern, removing the *problem story* and overlaying a new story with a therapeutic element to it which fills in the gaps we need to know so that we aren't stuck within the problem story.

How to Use These Stories?

There are many ways that these stories can be used. I gave a lot of thought to the best way to present them, whether to present them to be read at bedtime, or as you would find them if you listened to them so that you can record them in your own voice and at a pace that is comfortable for yourself or perhaps for someone else to listen to. For other hypnotherapists, they can be used like scripts in therapy sessions to help clients to tackle anxiety, worry and stress.

The main reason for writing these stories down was for my *Dan Jones Hypnosis* YouTube channel subscribers. I have often been asked by my subscribers whether I would release books of my stories. It is common to get

Introduction

messages from people saying that they never make it to the end of any of the stories, they are always asleep long before the end and they would love to read the stories to know how they go and how they end. With this in mind, I decided that the best way to present these stories is as authentic as possible to how they are on YouTube.

If you decided to read these stories to help you sleep at night I recommend that you read them in a specific way. It is no good reading through a story fast, in an upbeat voice, or skim-reading. The two ways to read are either to read the stories exactly as they are written and where it talks about "listening to me" or "listening to my voice" you can interpret this to mean that inner voice you are using, *as if* you are listening to your inner voice talking to you. Alternatively, you can change these words and phrases to suit what you are doing, so that they match your ongoing experience. For example, instead of saying "as you listen to me and begin to drift comfortably asleep, I don't know whether you will find yourself drifting asleep more to the sound of my voice or the words I use, or perhaps to the spaces between my words.

And as you drift comfortably asleep I'll just tell a story in the background."

You would say to yourself "as I read this and begin to drift comfortably asleep, I don't know whether I will find myself drifting asleep more to the sound of my voice or the words I read, or perhaps to the spaces between the words. And as I drift comfortably asleep I'll just read this story to myself." (I will place this at the beginning of each story so that you can read it if you prefer).

As you read a story, you want to read slowly in a calm and relaxed voice, whether you do this in your head or out loud. You want to have plenty of pauses at times which feel comfortable and natural for you, often at full stops and shorter pauses at commas. Add additional calming emphasis when reading relaxing words and phrases like "begin to relax" and "deeper."

Remember, each story as presented by me on YouTube is between 20 minutes for the shortest of these stories, up to about 35 minutes in length for the longest stories. When reading these you want to read the stories at a slow and calm pace that takes a similar length of time.

Introduction

You want to read with few distractions, ideally when already in bed ready to fall asleep and with enough light to read by, but not too much light that it interferes with falling asleep.

There is a trick which will make the stories more effective while reading (I will place a summary of these three steps at the start of each story for ease of use):

- Before you read a story, think about what you want to achieve from reading it, for example "I want to fall asleep" and rate on a scale out of 1 to 10 how much you want to achieve this (10 being the most, 1 being the least).

- Then take a moment to think about something you have successfully achieved during the day. It doesn't matter what it is. It could be that you arrived at work on time, or successfully prepared dinner, or completed another task. Think fully about this experience, for a minute or two, thinking through what you did. So, if it was getting to work on time, you may think through the routine you went through to leave home with enough time to arrive at work on time, think about the journey and then think about arriving at work and noticing you were on time.

- Then tell yourself the intention "when I read this story (preferably name the story – like *Lake of Inner Discovery*), then I will fall asleep by the end of the story"

It is important to do these three things in this order and take them seriously before reading the story. The higher you genuinely scale that you want to fall asleep the more chance there is that you will fall asleep because the motivation to want to fall asleep from the story is higher, which gives greater strength to the intention to fall asleep from reading the story. You can alter the wording of the intention (stage 3) a little to suit what you want. You want to keep the "when I read this story, then…" but you can alter what comes after then. For example, it could be "then I will fall asleep as soon as I close this book" or "then I will fall asleep as soon as I turn off my Kindle" or "then I will fall asleep as soon as I finish this story" whatever it is that fits with your preference.

LAKE OF INNER DISCOVERY

Steps for increasing effectiveness of the story:

1. What do you want to achieve from reading this?

2. Think about one thing you have achieved today.

3. Say to yourself "When I read this story then…"

Alternative introduction:

"As I read this and begin to drift comfortably asleep, I don't know whether I will find myself drifting asleep more to the sound of my voice or the words I read, or perhaps to the spaces between the words. And as I drift comfortably asleep I'll just read this story to myself."

As you listen to me you can begin to relax and you will relax as deeply and comfortably as you can right now. And as the experience goes on, so you will relax deeper and even more comfortably. To the point where, as you continue listening to this adult bedtime story, you will discover yourself falling asleep without even noticing. And you will continue the story perhaps in your dreams, or perhaps you will get through to near the end of the story and just drift off asleep, deeply and comfortably, getting the appropriate sleep through the night.

And so, as you continue listening to me I'm going to tell you a story where you are the main character and it can be a little bit like a lucid dream where you are aware of the story playing out around you, aware of what you can see, what you can hear, what you can feel.

And so you go on a journey one day and as you take this journey, you are walking out through the woods and while you walk through the woods, you are wondering about different things, you are wondering about what it is you have got to do later, you are wondering about a conversation you had earlier or the previous day, you are wondering about someone you are going to see later in the week and a part of you is also aware of, the sounds around you, is also aware of the feeling of each footstep you take as you walk through the woods, is also aware of the sounds of the rustling leaves and noticing the dancing light, as it shimmers through the trees.

And while you are out on this nice and relaxed walk, you are searching for a lake, you have never visited this lake before, you have been told that if you come out into this wood you can discover a lake, a lake that will help you find some inner discovery and you are curious what inner discovery you can get by finding this lake. So, as you are out walking around you notice rabbits hopping around, you notice birds flying, you notice butterflies and bees going about their daily business; popping in and out of different flowers.

And you don't know what kind of inner discovery you are going to gain at the lake and what it is about the lake that will help you find that inner discovery, you just know it is what you have been told. So, you walk along the path going deeper into the woods and as you go deeper and deeper into the woods, so you relax more with the experience, that kind of daydream relaxation that you have, as you are walking along, where your mind is wandering and feeling pleasant, where the day just feels so pleasant, that you just feel so relaxed. And while you wander along you hear someone down the path, so you keep walking, you are curious who that person is going to be and as you get closer you can hear their voice speaking louder.

And then as you approach you notice, a man dressed in nondescript clothing, a man who can just blend in anywhere, he even seemed to almost blend in here, if it wasn't for his talking. And because you are walking through the woods and there is only you and this man, it is only polite to say hello, as you walk past. And as you walk past and you say hello, so the man responds to you. "Do you know where you are going here in the middle of nowhere?" The man asks.

You think you understand what the man says as you experience a little confusion and you tell him yes you are trying to find the lake and he responds "Yes you are trying to find the lake and the lake is in the middle of nowhere and nowhere is where you are going and you will know where you are going when you discover that nowhere is here and here in the middle of nowhere is nowhere. And some people try to travel to somewhere and other people try to travel to anywhere, but you're not trying to go somewhere or anywhere, you are here nowhere and as you walk around here nowhere, you should be able to find the lake you are looking for. Because the lake you are looking for is nowhere, but in your mind." And with that the man began to walk away. And left you feeling a little confused.

And so, you continued to walk along the path looking for the lake and you didn't know where you were going exactly, but you knew that you would find the lake following this path. So you continued looking along the path, going deeper into the woods and as you relax deeper and deeper into the woods, so the, woods appear to, become thicker and denser and that made them become slightly darker, but that helped you to notice that as you turned a corner on the path, that there was a clearing off in the distance because it was much brighter over there and you didn't pick up the pace or speed up in anyway just because you noticed the clearing, but you now knew where you were going. You were confident that in that clearing, that you would find the lake that you were searching for. And as you are walking along towards that clearing, so you have the words of that man going around in your head. Nowhere, somewhere, anywhere. You thought to yourself quizzically. Nowhere, somewhere, anywhere.

You didn't know exactly what he was on about, but the same way when you meet someone and you can't remember their name but you know you know their name but the harder you try to remember their name, the harder it becomes to remember and then you just put it out of your mind and you carry on with other things and then their name springs up in your mind a little while later, you knew the same thing would probably happy here and if you just carry on with the journey and you put what that man said out of your mind and the answer will just spring up in mind when the time is right, there is no need to try and force it, the answers will come through when the unconscious has worked it out enough to let you know.

And as you approach the clearing you notice the most beautiful lake, such calm water and as you gaze across the lake the water is so calm that the reflection in the water is almost indistinguishable from what it is reflecting. And you are aware that if you took a photo and turned the photo upside-down people probably wouldn't be able to tell which one is the water and which one is the sky, which one is just the reflection.

And you had never seen a lake as still as this and you felt it was really odd that this lake should be so still given there was the most refreshing, beautiful breeze on your skin. Because you expect the breeze to move the water.

And as you approach the lake you can see a sign and so you walk over to the sign and on the sign, is some writing and the writing says 'pick up a stone and throw it in and watch how it sinks to the bottom and keep your eyes firmly fixed on the stone, don't be distracted by the ripples of the lake, don't be distracted by any other movement, don't be distracted by sounds, just keep your eyes focused on the stone as it hits the water and sinks to the bottom and keep your eyes focused on that stone and you will gain inner discovery.'

And then there was an arrow pointing down beneath the sign to some purple stones. And next to the purple stones was a small sign, saying 'pick the stone that feels right for you' and so you put your hand down and you feel the different stones and you can feel how some are rougher than others and you can see that some were matt and others are reflective and you can see how the stones are all different shapes and sizes. They all have different textures and so you feel the different stones in your fingertips, feeling the weight, the size, the shape, until you find one that feels right and comfortable for you.

And once you have found that comfortable stone you can throw it in the lake and you can let your eyes follow the stone through the air as it arches towards the lake. You let your eyes follow the stone to the surface, hearing that sound of the stone breaking the surface, seeing the splash of water, hearing the plop sound as the stone enters the lake and watching as the stone waves slightly left and right as it sinks to the bottom and as the sign said, you keep your eyes on the stone as it sinks to the bottom and while it is on the bottom you keep your eyes on the stone and you notice how the ripples begin to spread out from where the stone entered the water and as the ripples reach the shore, so the reeds by the bank begin to wave as they are knocked about by the water. And as the ripples travel across the lake so they spread out further and further. Spreading further apart as they travel across the lake and you followed the instructions, you have kept your eyes focused and fixed on that stone, out of your peripheral vision you can notice the movement and you don't let it bother you, you just keep your eyes fixed on the stone and after a few minutes the strangest thing can begin to happen. Your peripheral vision begins to go black and the stone begins to become even clearer and you begin to have a sense of clarity.

And then as the lake becomes still, you notice that between you and the stone is you and it is as if you are looking into your own eyes, looking into your own soul, looking into your heart. Seeing yourself for the first time. Not the self you normally see in a mirror, but your deeper self, your inner self. And so you can take some time of peace and silence, feeling a slight sense of excitement of your discovery, to begin to, gain that inner discovery, from the weird reflective nature of this lake and how that is somehow connected to a stone entering the lake, creating ripples yet everything becomes still like nothing has happened and yet you are aware something has happened, you are aware, something entered the lake and the lake is different to how it was before you arrived because of your actions and yet on the surface it looks no different, but deep down, something has changed and so you take some time to enjoy some silence to develop inner meaning and discovery.

And after a while, you feel you have been discovering something and learning something, deep inside your mind and so you begin to walk away from the lake. You now know where it is when you want to come back here again and so you walk away from the lake, back through the woods. And as you walk back through the woods so you walk deeper and deeper and drift deeper and deeper and fall asleep comfortably, easily and effortlessly. And you can take as long as you like to absorb yourself in the process of walking back through the woods and knowing unconsciously there is a lot that you have learned. And so, you can enjoy taking a nice leisurely stroll back through the woods, going deeper and more comfortably asleep.

The Astronaut's Wonder

Steps for increasing effectiveness of the story:

1. What do you want to achieve from reading this?

2. Think about one thing you have achieved today.

3. Say to yourself "When I read this story then…"

Alternative introduction:

"As I read this and begin to drift comfortably asleep, I don't know whether I will find myself drifting asleep more to the sound of my voice or the words I read, or perhaps to the spaces between the words. And as I drift comfortably asleep I'll just read this story to myself."

As you listen to this, so you will begin to fall asleep and you may fall asleep before the end of this or you may feel comfortably relaxed and drift off into a comfortable sleep at the end of this and as you listen to this, this also has useful therapeutic messages within this story and it's not a detailed story, it's purpose is to be a bit like drifting in a dream where you are playing the lead role, where it is something calming and comfortable, that helps you drift comfortably asleep.

So as you listen to me, you can begin to notice yourself as an astronaut. You are walking along towards a giant rocket and you have got some astronaut crew with you. You are all walking along towards that giant rocket. You look down at yourself and see the suit that you are wearing and you are carrying the helmet at the moment and you feel the weight of the suit and perhaps you can be surprised that the suit isn't as hot as you expected it to be for something that is so big and so heavy and surprised that you can move so easily in the suit. And you see people taking photos of you and your fellow astronauts as you walk towards the rocket and you can see the clear blue sky above you, feel the warmth of the sun, smelling the fresh air, hearing the murmuring sounds of the people, feeling a little bit in awe of the size of that rocket as you get closer to it and realising how small you appear next to it. And as you get closer to the rocket, so you and your fellow astronauts enter a lift that takes you up what looks like scaffolding up to the height of the entrance to the rocket and you let some of the other astronauts go first and then you walk out behind them and you admire the view from being so high up and you think to yourself that it is like standing at the top of the Eiffel Tower and you walk along the platform and you can hear the echoey metallic sound of each step you take and you enter the shuttle, closing the door behind you, hearing the sound of the door closing and you can feel the weight of the door as you close the door, although you can feel the door is heavy, it feels surprisingly smooth and manoeuvrable and moves with ease and you get into your seat and put your helmet on and twist it slightly to lock it in place and you can notice how you can now hear your breathing from within your helmet and notice how different the breathing sounds now breathing inside the helmet and you strap yourself in and think to yourself how awkward it is getting into the seat and strapping yourself in, when you are having to climb into the seat and lift your legs up, almost like sitting in a seat that is lying on its back.

Then you hear mission control begin to count down. They let you know everything is okay, the checks have all been done, we are safe for take-off, then they begin to count down, 10, 9, 8 and as they count down, your mind begins to focus, 7, 6, 5, 4, 3 and at three you hear a rumbling as the burners are lit, 2 and you hear a rumbling coming from the rockets, 1, 0 and on the count of zero, there is a moments pause and then suddenly what feels like an earthquake around you, a rumbling, tumbling earthquake, if there were things that could rattle you know they would. And you feel like you are lifting and you don't quite recognise it as lifting and you can't see anything outside other than a little bit of blue sky and so you can't notice that you are lifting and then after a second or two suddenly you start to feel really heavy and find yourself pushed back in your seat and after five seconds you feel like you have tripled in weight. And the rocket continues to accelerate and it quickly breaks the speed of sound and all of a sudden

The Astronaut's Wonder

there is silence from outside, as you are travelling faster than the sound is able to travel from the rockets to your ears.

The acceleration continues, the sky begins to get darker and darker outside and you are aware that you must be rising up higher and higher in the earth's atmosphere. After about 15 seconds, you begin to, notice yourself becoming weightless. Suddenly the shuttle twists and turns. Out of the window you see the earth. Like a giant blue marble in space. You enjoy in awe, the view, gazing down at the earth, as the shuttle begins to circle the earth. And you unbuckle yourself and notice how you are weightless and everything just floats. And you explore the shuttle. And this isn't an ordinary shuttle, this is the latest shuttle, for a new kind of trip to space.

Part of your role in space, is to go and do a spacewalk. You have got to take a specific satellite out of the shuttle with you, just a small satellite and you have got to unfurl its solar panels, attach a few pieces to it and do all that far enough away from the shuttle, that there is no risk to the shuttle or to the satellite. And so, you leave the shuttle on your spacewalk. And you work on sorting out that satellite and you wonder what the satellite is for. You know it is to help with communication but you don't know in what context. And it is hard work to work on the satellite, but you enjoy it because you are out in space. While you are working on the satellite, a part of your mind is wondering about how in space there is no up nor down, no left, nor right, no backwards or forwards, there just *is*. You are aware that to you, you feel like you are stationary, sorting out a satellite, you can notice that the earth is moving beneath you, but you don't feel like you are moving. And yet you are aware that you are actually travelling around the earth at thousands of miles per hour. And you are aware that you are ageing at a different speed to your family back on earth. And so you start to ponder what reality is, if you can be travelling at thousands of miles per hour and feel like you are stationary and if you can be ageing slower than family on earth.

Once you have sorted the satellite out, you let go of it, having pressed in some codes and it autocorrects, gets itself to the correct orbit and you head back to the shuttle. Then the shuttle has a few days of orbiting the earth, where you do a few science experiments and relax, you take photos of the night sky, you take photos of the earth, you get a new perspective on things from up here, you learn and grow and after a few days in space, it is time for you to return back to earth. As you buckle back into the shuttle, the trajectory of the shuttle is changed. You begin to make the journey back down into the earth's atmosphere and as you journey back down into the earth's atmosphere, so you journey deeper asleep. You feel so relaxed journeying down into the earth's atmosphere, aware of how well built the shuttle is, how successful the shuttle is landing. Being able to enjoy the journey back down, noticing how the blackness of space starts to change to a blue of the atmosphere, passing through layers of cloud, before heading for a giant runway, landing on that runway, firing parachutes out the back of the shuttle to decelerate the shuttle and being welcomed home, almost like a hero's welcome, because, although space flight is now more common, it is still not something everyone does all the time. And you can look forward to your next space flight, to the next time you get called upon to repair a satellite, to take a satellite into space. And you can drift comfortably asleep now.

A Lesson in Harmony

Steps for increasing effectiveness of the story:

1. What do you want to achieve from reading this?
2. Think about one thing you have achieved today.
3. Say to yourself "When I read this story then…"

Alternative introduction:

"As I read this and begin to drift comfortably asleep, I don't know whether I will find myself drifting asleep more to the sound of my voice or the words I read, or perhaps to the spaces between the words. And as I drift comfortably asleep I'll just read this story to myself."

So, as you listen to me and begin to drift comfortably asleep, I don't know whether you will find yourself drifting asleep more to the sound of my voice or the words I use, or perhaps to the spaces between my words. And as you drift comfortably asleep I'll just tell a story in the background.

This person went to the same café every day, it was part of their routine, they enjoyed going out, getting out of home for a while, going for a little walk and wandering down this cobbled street that is quite a quiet street and a bit of a back street, somewhere where there weren't too many people, to this independent café. And they enjoyed going into that café. Sitting down at a table, drinking their favourite drink and relaxing and they could spend a while in this café, just sitting down, drinking their favourite drink, relaxing, while watching out the window, watching people walking past, going about their daily business, in their own little worlds, hearing the sounds of the coffee maker and other sounds in the café and the clinking of china and metal teaspoons. And the mumble, mumble sounds of voices in the background, unable to make out any one voice, or word, or sentence, but just having this mumbling sound of other people in the background. Finding it all deeply relaxing. And while finding it all deeply relaxing, they often find their mind begins to wander and as their mind begins to wander they discover themselves gently stirring their drink, gazing at a rose in a vase on their table. And as they gaze at that rose in that vase on their table, so everything else begins to fade away. They stop being aware of the sounds around them, they stop being aware of people walking past outside. Everything begins to fade away as their attention is absorbed on that rose and while their attention is absorbed on that rose, so they begin to drift and dream, they begin to drift into a pleasant reverie.

And they enjoy just letting what happens, happen, as they drift comfortably inside and while they gaze at that rose, first they notice how that rose begins to grow, begins to start getting taller and wider, getting taller and wider and taller and wider and as that rose continues to get taller and wider, so they notice it begins to spread wider than the vase, breaking the vase, then it gets wider and wider, taller and taller and they notice that at some point it merges and morphs into a tree trunk and the top of the rose begins to fall away and spread out and merge into a trees canopy and as this all happens, so the café around them begins to fade away and disappear. And they find themselves sitting in what looks like a monastery on that café chair with no table in front of them anymore and no café surrounding them anymore. Instead they have got a stone wall off a little way in the distance that goes along in front of them and then turns and goes along beside them and then some way off it turns again and goes off back behind them.

When they look the other way they notice there is a monastery there and there are people quietly milling around in the monastery, walking with purpose, walking slowly. Almost as if it is taking them no effort. And then as they bring their eyes back to looking in front of them they notice how the tree has stopped growing and the chair they thought they were sitting on moments ago is now a stone bench.

And they stand up gently from that stone bench. They reach over and touch the tree, they feel how real that tree feels. They walk around the tree running their hand around the bark. Feeling the reality of that tree. Continuing to walk around while looking up at the canopy, noticing the way the sun dances and twinkles through the leaves and noticing the way the leaves move in the breeze. Noticing the reality of the experience. And they walk over to the stone wall and the stone wall is slightly lower than they are at points and they walk over to one of the lower points and they look out over the stone wall and see that they are part way up a hill and that they can see down the bottom of the hill that there is a road that leads all the way down there and what looks like a village down there with people with stalls selling fruit and veg and other things.

And they take a deep breath of the air and can smell how different the air is here. And they start carefully walking around the monastery and as they walk around so they meet one of the people in the monastery who tells them to walk with intent. And they think to themselves, they were walking with intent, they decided to walk and they were walking slowly like everyone else. And they were told they were walking slowly to copy others and they knew they wanted to walk but they weren't walking with intent, they weren't just focusing on the walking, their mind was elsewhere. And this person taught them about walking focusing on the walking, about being focused on the one thing you are doing in any one moment and paying that one thing your full attention, not living in the future all the time, not living in the past all the time, not living else where all the time, but being grounded, being present here. And they told the person to reach down and touch the ground with their fingertips and the person thought this was a bit of an odd request but they felt comfortable doing this and so they reached down and touched the grass and they were asked "What do you feel?".

They replied that they feel the grass. And they were told "No, look inside yourself, what do you feel?".

And they thought about it and they thought about it and they started to feel a connection with the earth, they started to feel the grass on a deeper level, they started to feel like they were connected with the grass, not something separate from the grass. And the person turned with intent and started walking away with one hand behind their back. And this person started following them. And as they followed, that person started walking in this direction and then that direction and seemed to be just walking for the sake of walking. And then they stopped. And they turned and they spoke again. And they asked "What are you doing?".

And the person said "I was just following you, to learn from you.".

And they explained that they didn't need to be followed, that all they have done is led them all over the place, nothing is meaningful, none of the movement was meaningful. And the person said "But, you seemed so wise I thought if I followed you I could learn from you and you could teach me some of your wisdom.".

And they said "You don't want to learn my wisdom by following me, you want to learn wisdom by looking inside yourself and your connection to the world around you, not by following someone else.".

And the person then turned and walked away and this time, they weren't followed. And the person thought to themselves "This is a long way from the café." as they explored the monastery.

And while exploring the monastery they wondered if they would be allowed inside. They walked over to the door and they knocked on the door, the door was opened and the person who opened it stepped aside and didn't talk to them. And they walked in and started exploring the inside of the monastery. And nobody got in their way, nobody told them they couldn't look anywhere, they seemed to be allowed to roam wherever they wanted, supposedly there was full trust of them.

They explored around the monastery, they noticed that everything was very simple and everyone seemed so peaceful, so calm and relaxed. And they walked around the monastery and then up some stairs, they found a spiral staircase and they followed that staircase up to the next floor, they explored this floor, they saw rooms for sleeping and yet every bed was really simple. Everything just seemed to be practical and serve a purpose. And they gazed out of a window from up here, they looked out and could see the town, they could see off into the distance, all the way over to some distant forest. They could see clouds in the sky.

They then walked up another spiral staircase, going higher up into the monastery and then they found a wooden door, they opened the wooden door and found themselves on the rooftop. They decided to walk out onto the roof and explore. They were taken aback by the view from up here and the fresh air, they gazed out over the view, they kept walking around and gazed out over the view from different directions and as they turned around their heart skipped a beat when they saw a huge dragon resting in the middle of the rooftop. They felt a bit nervous and anxious about this dragon, they started trying to creep around, not wanting to wake the dragon, not wanting to be seen by the dragon, worried that maybe the dragon would eat them or breathe fire on them. The dragon noticed them, opened its eyes, jolted up its head, stood up and looked even larger. Moved its neck and its head down almost nose to nose with the person. And the breathing, the breath, could be felt as well as heard. Bursts of powerful breath. And the dragon just watched with its head ever so slightly in front of the person's head and the person moved sideways and the dragon held their gaze and the person moved back the other direction and the dragon held their gaze and the person stood still.... and the dragon held their gaze. The person didn't know what to think, was the dragon about to attack? Why was the dragon not doing anything, just holding their gaze? And after a while of the dragon holding their gaze their nervousness began to decrease because they didn't know whether they should be nervous or not, they didn't know what was going on. And as their nervousness decreased, so the dragon lowered its head and rested its head down on the ground, still maintaining eye contact and as the nervousness decreased further the dragon sat itself down, still maintaining eye contact. And the more the dragon looked calm and relaxed the more the person relaxed themselves and as the person relaxed deeper, so the dragons breathing seemed to relax deeper.

And then they felt this compulsion to walk along the side of the dragon to touch the dragons neck to feel what the dragons skin feels like. And as they touched the dragon's neck the dragon just remained there calm and relaxed and they moved their hand along the dragon's neck as they walked along towards its body and as they reached the dragons body it lowered its nearest wing as if to say "climb aboard" and the person had this feeling, that was what the dragon was trying to tell them.

So they climbed up onto the dragons back and with incredibly fast reflexes the dragon just leapt off the top of the monastery up into the air and the person grabbed on tight and the dragon started flying and the person had this sense of being thrown all around, not like the dragon was trying to hurt them, but like they just weren't used to this experience, like being in a fighter jet. And as the dragon flew around and did different aerobatics, the person began to fall into synch with the dragon, to get in tune with the dragon, began to feel a sense of harmony and when the dragon banked left the person knew to lean and when the dragon banked right, the person knew to lean and the person learned to respond to subtler and subtler communication, knowing when to lean just at the moment they needed to lean. And the more they fell into harmony with the dragon the calmer and more relaxed they felt and the more they enjoyed the experience.

And then after a long time of flying around on the dragon, the dragon flew back to the monastery, crashed down onto the monastery, landing with a thud, dropped its head, its neck, its legs, lowered its wings and the person climbed off the dragon's back, feeling serene, feeling a sense of wonder, a sense of harmony with the dragon and now a sense of harmony with this land. As they walked back down the spiral staircase and then down the next spiral staircase, they left the monastery and they found that original person who they had followed around, who said "I see you have learned what you came here to learn, you understand what you needed to understand."

And they intuitively knew what this meant and they went back to the bench, sat back down on the stone bench, gazing at the tree, resting their hands on their legs, breathing deep and comfortably and as they did, with each breath out, so the tree began to shrink back down again and began to turn back into a rose. And as that tree shrunk down and turned into a rose, so the vase repaired itself around the rose, the table appeared again, the outside world appeared again and the café appeared again. And the chair they were sitting on was the café chair again. And they instinctively found their hand lift off of their leg and continue stirring that drink and they realised the reverie had come to an end and that they were back in the café with the mumbling background sounds of the people, sounds of the coffee maker, the clinking of china and spoons, people walking past outside and no-one aware that this experience had happened, but them. And they knew that later that night they would go home and they would probably continue to process this learning when they sleep and dream.

A Relaxing Break

Steps for increasing effectiveness of the story:

1. What do you want to achieve from reading this?

2. Think about one thing you have achieved today.

3. Say to yourself "When I read this story then…"

Alternative introduction:

"As I read this and begin to drift comfortably asleep, I don't know whether I will find myself drifting asleep more to the sound of my voice or the words I read, or perhaps to the spaces between the words. And as I drift comfortably asleep I'll just read this story to myself."

Bedtime Stories for Grown-ups

As you begin to comfortably drift asleep I don't know whether you will find yourself drifting comfortably asleep faster to the sound of my voice or perhaps to the words I use, or maybe you will drift asleep faster to the spaces between my words and as you fall asleep I will just be telling a story in the background and while I tell the story you can just drift asleep comfortably.

And there was a woman sitting by a campfire on a beach and the sun was setting on the horizon, the sky was a beautiful orange and red and looking in the other direction she could see the dark blue gradually stretching across the sky, she could notice how some stars were beginning to appear, as that sun continued to set. She could see the way the water was gently lapping on the shore and hear the sound of that gentle lapping on the shore. She could feel the warmth from the sand as it hadn't yet radiated away all of the warmth from the days sun. And found her attention drawn to, the flickering and dancing of the campfire flame. She was sat here with her wife, the two of them had come out on a trip to camp on the beach. To enjoy some time relaxing. A break away from real-life, a break away from the hustle and bustle of everything you normally have to get up to and do and instead, slow things down and relax.

As the sun continued to set, so they huddled up closer to each other to keep warm around that fire while just talking and gazing out over the sea, watching as more stars appear in the sky. And then once the sun had fully set over the horizon and the sky was beginning to turn a dark and inky blue, they laid on their backs gazing up at the stars, wondering with curiosity about what might be out there, talking about different things, watching the occasional shooting star go over. Watching as they see little dots travelling across the sky, aware that these are satellites and wondering which satellites they are seeing. Noticing the flashing lights of planes passing overhead. And occasionally hearing the sound of the planes. And discussing how curious it is, the way that the sound of the plane clearly sounds like it comes from a different location to where you can see the plane, because of the difference in the speed of sound and the speed of light. And how curious it is that you don't normally notice that in everyday life, in conversations, it is only when things are over a slightly longer distance that you notice that, what you see and what you hear are things that happen at two different times. And they start talking about how this would be the case if there was a thunderstorm on the horizon, they would see the lightning dancing in the sky and it would take a while before they hear the thunder reach their ears.

And they talk about how it is interesting that in most movies, these things are synchronised even though in reality they wouldn't be. They talk about how in movies you can see an explosion happen and the sight and the sound of the explosion happen at the same time, even if the character viewing the explosion is some distance away. And it is interesting, that despite it being natural, it feels unnatural when you see this in a movie. And that very few movies seem to keep this natural.

And they always found that they did this, that whenever they had time to relax, time away from work, from other commitments, they would talk about all of these things, the things that individually they think about, but never really share with anyone else. And gradually as the night drew on and got darker and darker the two of them pulled a blanket up over themselves and snuggled down

A Relaxing Break

and fell asleep for the night and then in the morning, they had already planned what they were going to do, they were going to start the day with an early morning meditation on the beach before going for a walk in the nearby woods and then coming back to the beach afterwards to have something to eat and to settle down for an evening again.

And so, the two of them stood on the sand barefoot so that they could feel the sand beneath their feet and through their toes and they stood up and closed their eyes and started focusing on breathing in and breathing out. They started focusing on making each "out" breath longer than each "in" breath so that they would trigger the relaxation response and then they started using their senses, paying attention to the world around them, they focused outside of themselves, firstly on the sea, on the rhythmic way the waves washed ashore and the way the waves pulled back out to sea and then washed ashore again and then pulled back out to sea. They focused on the sounds of the waves and in their minds eye they started to see the waves and feel the waves; to really honestly and fully experience those waves in their mind.

They then focused their attention on the sounds of birds, the sounds of birds above them and off in the distance and then focused on the feeling of the breeze on their face and their skin, working out the direction of the breeze, noticing the temperature of the breeze, noticing the difference between the temperature of the breeze and the temperature of their skin, noticing the way the breeze blew their hair.

And they focused on their body, on what their body felt like standing there and on the smell of the salty air and they allowed themselves to be drawn in to the moment, drawn in to the experience. And then after a while, about fifteen minutes that seemed like a couple of hours they both came around from their meditation, they took a little while to sit down to have a bit of a chat before setting off into the woods. They then set off into the woods to go on a walk, they listened to the animals in the woods, they watched the way that rays of light penetrate the canopy and dance in front of them, they notice how being in the woods subdued some of the sound making things that little bit quieter. And after a little while they could no longer hear the sound of the sea, they could barely hear the sound of birds outside of the woods and they walked deeper and deeper into the woods.

After a little while walking deeper into the woods they found a clearing and in that clearing was a lake and sat on a rock beside the lake was a little bluey-purpley creature and it looked so friendly and kind and so they walked over to it and they spoke to it and they asked it who it was and what it was doing here and the creature said its name was Moz and that it is just a friendly creature just relaxing here looking over the lake waiting for anyone to talk to, anyone to share some kindness with. And they were told that if they walk around the lake they will find a cabin and inside the cabin is a secret door and behind that secret door is a secret room and in that secret room is a secret drink and next to the secret drink is a book explaining about the drink.

They wondered why they were being told this? They were told that they were the first people who have come along here in a very, very long time and they seem kind and caring people, they seem calm and relaxed people and everyone deserves to be treated with kindness and that is all that is happening here. They thanked the creature and discussed with each other that perhaps they will go searching for that cabin. So, they started walking around the lake, the woods on one side and the lake on the other side and the gentle lapping of the water on the shore of the lake, the rustling of the leaves in the woods of the breeze, the feeling of the warmth of the sun and the sounds of their footsteps as they walked around trying to find that cabin.

After sometime walking around the lake they found the cabin they assumed had been talked about. They knocked on the door. No-one answered. They walked into the cabin. Inside the cabin it was cosy and relaxing. It seemed such a friendly place to be. They sat down for a while having walked all this way. While they were sat down they were looking around the inside of the cabin, aware that somewhere here was a secret door. After a little while they stood up and started to check around the walls, they started to move books on the bookshelves, they started to move ornaments, anything which looked like it could be a button or lever, they would move it, yet nothing seemed to open anything.

A Relaxing Break

Then one of them walked across a rug in front of the fireplace and as they did they noticed that the sound of their footsteps changed, not just because they walked onto the rug, they noticed that their footsteps had changed because perhaps underneath the rug was a secret door. They moved the rug and saw a hatchway, they opened the hatch and saw a ladder. They climbed down the ladder and found themselves deep under the cabin in a secret room.

They turned on the light in this secret room and in the middle of the room was a book on a pedestal and next to the book was a drink. They walked over and opened the book and started to read the book. Reading that under this spot is a spring, a spring that heals. And that the water here has this healing property that rejuvenates cells, that heals outwardly from the cells and it went on to explain how it worked, what the theories were behind it. It went on to explain the history of those who lived here. It explained about how they had ended up building a cabin over this space, it was a cabin over a cavern.

They looked at each other and wondered whether they should drink this drink or not. They decided to just have a sip or two each and see what happens and they drunk some of the drink each and could feel the coolness of that water passing down through their bodies, then they could feel this sensation, like healing happening, passing through their body, starting to pass around their body, as if this healing was getting right into each and every cell of their body, right down into their genes. And they felt this profound healing take place.

After experiencing this profound healing they left the cabin, started their way back along the edge of the lake, they met the creature again who smiled and said they could tell they have had the drink and that if there was anything wrong within their body, that healing drink will have sorted that out, would have searched for it and healed those areas, helping to rejuvenate them and reset them back so that all of the cells were as they should be, as the cells memories say they should be. They carried on through the woods, back to that beach where they sat down on the beach and settled down for the night and once again they enjoyed watching as the sun set and the stars rose and appeared, as they drifted comfortably relaxed asleep in each other's arms.

THE SCULPTURE INSIGHT

Steps for increasing effectiveness of the story:

1. What do you want to achieve from reading this?

2. Think about one thing you have achieved today.

3. Say to yourself "When I read this story then…"

Alternative introduction:

"As I read this and begin to drift comfortably asleep, I don't know whether I will find myself drifting asleep more to the sound of my voice or the words I read, or perhaps to the spaces between the words. And as I drift comfortably asleep I'll just read this story to myself."

So as you listen to me and you begin to comfortably fall asleep, I don't know whether you will fall asleep quicker with the sound of my voice, or with the words that I use, or perhaps with the spaces between my words and as you begin to comfortably fall asleep I'm just going to tell you a story in the background and it is a story about a man who is sitting on a beach, it is a nice warm sunny day and the beach is quite quiet and he has come here to sit down and relax. And while he is sitting on the beach he is reading a book and as he is reading so his attention is being drawn into that book, drawn into the story and in the background he is aware that there is the sound of the waves lashing on the shore, aware of the sounds of birds in the sky, he is aware of distant sounds around him, he can feel the warmth of the sun on his face, he can feel what the ground feels like beneath him where he is sitting and yet his attention is drawn into the book.

And while he is reading the book, he finds that it is almost like the story jumps off the page and starts to form in his mind. As if, he starts off reading and hearing the words recited in his own voice in his mind and then gradually that reciting voice fades away to almost experiencing the story on the page and the story that he is reading is about someone out on a boat and they are heading to an island and the boat is bobbing up and down on the water and chugging through the water and it is a warm sunny day, while this boat is chugging through the water. There is blue sky, perhaps some wispy clouds, but it is a warm sunny day and as that boat continues, so the man on the boat notices the island coming into view in the distance. And continues on that boat towards that island and the boat continues to move with the waves, as well as moving through the waves.

On arrival near the island there is nowhere to dock the boat. So, the man drops anchor a little way from the island, lowers down a rigid inflatable boat off of the back of his boat into the water, climbs aboard that boat and powers towards the shore. This smaller boat, jumps and bounces on the waves as it nears the shore. The man cuts the engine and glides the boat up onto the beach. Here on the island he can hear the sounds of tropical birds, the way the water laps onto the sand, the sound of the sand beneath his feet. And he starts exploring the island.

He is here to discover something and as he explores the island, he finds a beachball that appears to have been washed up here. And almost instinctively he picks up the beachball, just to carry that beachball and to play with that beachball in his hands, he doesn't know why, it just seems to be an instinctive thing, he just saw it and picked it up and walked along tossing it gently into the air, spinning it slightly in the air, noticing the vivid, bold colours on that beachball as he throws it, catches it and spins it while he is exploring the island.

He cuts into the trees, works his way through the trees and as the trees get denser he has to put down the beachball to continue, so that he can push through those trees. And after a while he finds himself on the far side of this island, on a different beach. And on this side of the island he notices that the water is far rougher, the waves are far higher, he can see dark clouds out to sea and the occasional flash of lightning on the horizon, although it is too far to hear any rumbles of thunder. And he starts exploring this side of the island, starts exploring this beach. He doesn't know exactly what he is looking for but he knows he will recognise it when he finds it.

And after some time exploring, he sees what looks like part of a chest poking out from the sand and he goes over and with his hands he digs around the chest until he can pull the chest out of the sand and onto the beach.

He breaks the lock open and opens the chest. Inside the chest he finds a book. While sat down next to the chest he starts flicking through the pages of that book, starts reading the pages of the book and looking at the images in that book. And realises that it is teaching him some kind of knowledge, something he has to do. And that it is going to take a long time to do it. He realises that this column of stone which is next to where he found the chest, that is just off the tree line, is there for a reason. He reads that he needs to carve a specific sculpture if he is to get what it is that he seeks. He reads in the book what that sculpture is supposed to look like, what carving he is supposed to do. In the chest, he sees that there is a hammer and chisel. He takes the hammer and chisel and starts chipping away at that stone, chipping away carefully in small amounts at a time, chipping away what isn't necessary, with the idea that it will leave just that which is necessary and he chips away and he chips away, as the day wears on and the sun starts to set.

He then sets up a camp on the beach for the night, lights a fire and has something to eat, falls asleep in a makeshift tent to the sounds of the water on the shore and the sight of millions of stars in the sky. The next morning after having something to eat he carries on chipping away at that stone, chipping away, carving and removing what isn't necessary, to leave what is essential. He continues to chip and carve away and by the middle of the day he begins to notice what is forming. He notices that it is starting to look like a person. He carries on chipping away and chipping away for the rest of the day and then settles down again for the night, before carrying on again the next morning. And he does this for a number of days and nights, chipping away at the sculpture, removing what isn't necessary and leaving that which is essential.

After a number of days of chipping away, he finally finishes the sculpture and sees that it looks like a person facing into the woods. But, he doesn't seem to have got what it is that he came here for. So, he doesn't fully understand. He has invested a lot of time and energy into chipping away at this sculpture and he sits down on the beach wondering what he is supposed to have learned, wondering what all of this means. He has removed all of that stone and yet this sculpture is just a sculpture of a person, it hasn't taught him anything. He has something to eat and he falls asleep that night wondering what this could all mean and he tries to let his brain process that, let his brain work on what this could all mean. He processes the last few days, processes the effort he has taken, all the information he has read. He was somehow supposed to gain knowledge from this, something that enriches your life, but he hasn't seen any treasures and he can't figure out the clue.

During his dream, he starts to have unusual thoughts, thoughts of being too warm and taking off some layers, of being too cold and putting new layers on. Thoughts of getting to know a best friend, or a loved one. By the morning, he awoke having an idea about what it is he was supposed to have learned from carving this sculpture and from chipping away all that material and leaving only that which is necessary for the sculpture.

He realises that this whole journey wasn't about gaining some kind of financial incentive, it was about enriching the inner life and learning about yourself and gaining a deep knowledge about yourself, about who you are, who you want to be, how you are and how you want to be and how to get from who you are and how you are, to who you want to be and how. He realised that was what working on this sculpture had taught him. That was the insight he was supposed to gain.

As he looked at the sculpture having gained that insight, just like a snowman the sculpture seemed to melt into nothing. Almost like it was built out of sand and the sand had just collapsed to the ground merging in with the rest of the sand. He placed the book back in the chest and he reburied the chest and prepared for a journey back home. He cut back through the trees, all the way back to the beach he arrived on. Pushed his boat into the water, started the motor, travelled back to his boat, got on his boat, raised his small boat, lifted the anchor and set off homeward. And as the story ended the man closed the book aware that he had learned something about himself from this story that he had decided to read.

And while he mindfully processed that story he stood up from the beach, walked down to the shore, could feel the way the sand went from dry and grainy to damp and stodgy where his feet would sink slightly into the sand with each step. He could see the area of dryness spread from under his foot each time he placed his foot down as it compressed the sand and pushed the water out of the way. And he noticed with each step that as he raised his foot that water rushed back in again making that sand damp again. And he walked to the water's edge and he walked a little way into the water and he could feel that the sea water was warm and he could feel the movement of the water around his ankles and his feet, the way it pulled the sand in and out that he could feel through his toes, he took a few deep breaths of sea air and could feel the warmth of the sun on his face as he enjoyed and processed the insights he had gained from reading that story and allowing himself to become absorbed in that story. He processed those insights as he just listened to the natural world around him and learned about who he is and how he is in this world, what his purpose is. Those parts of him he likes and those parts of him he would like to change and shift and who he would like to be and he learned from that sculpture.

After spending some time allowing all that to integrate, he then started travelling home, still thinking about how he is integrating all of this new learning. On arrival home, he had something to eat, he relaxed for a while, before going up to bed, closing his eyes and drifting deeply and comfortably asleep. And as he drifted comfortably asleep he began to dream about being on that island, about running his hands around the sculpture, feeling the handy work that was done, feeling a connection with that work, admiring that sculpture, learning from that sculpture, feeling the smoothness of the stone to the backdrop of a distant storm as the waves lashed on the shore and he felt himself drawn deeper and deeper into this healing dream as he drifted and floated deeper and deeper asleep, internalising and understanding this in a whole new level previously unknown, learning on an instinctive level, until his dream began to fade and he began to just drift even deeper and comfortably asleep.

THE STUDENT'S DREAM

Steps for increasing effectiveness of the story:

1. What do you want to achieve from reading this?

2. Think about one thing you have achieved today.

3. Say to yourself "When I read this story then…"

Alternative introduction:

"As I read this and begin to drift comfortably asleep, I don't know whether I will find myself drifting asleep more to the sound of my voice or the words I read, or perhaps to the spaces between the words. And as I drift comfortably asleep I'll just read this story to myself."

As you take a moment to close your eyes, you can begin to comfortably fall asleep and while you are comfortably falling asleep I don't know whether you will fall asleep faster with the sound of my voice, with the words that I use or whether you will fall asleep faster to the spaces between my words. And as you comfortably drift off to sleep, I'm going to tell a story in the background.

It is a story about a teenager who was in a library and this teenager is supposed to be studying and while they are turning the pages of a complex book they find that their mind isn't really in it. They are struggling to focus on the pages, they are struggling to take in what it is that they are studying. So, they decide that they are going to put some music on, they are going to listen to some music through headphones to help them to be able to focus on studying.

So, they put their headphones on, turn on their music and start to listen to some calming, relaxing music. And their headphones are noise-cancelling, so as the music begins, the noises around them fade away. There weren't many noises in the library anyway, but when you are trying to study, sometimes every little thing can catch your attention and prevent you from focusing and so you just need to alter the environment to one that helps you learn. So, they listen to their favourite music and as they do, while listening to that favourite relaxing music, their shoulders relax, their breathing starts to comfortably slow down and they notice their gaze changing, their facial muscles relaxing. They notice themselves starting to fall into a comfortable rhythm with reading and learning and they know that this strategy works well for them for studying, that what they can do is, during an exam, they can recall a piece of music and when they do, because learning is state-dependant, it re-evokes the state and all of the memories and learning that was done in that state. So, they listen to the music, gaze at the pages and find that somehow the learning is just comfortably going into their mind. As if they are easily and effortlessly learning one page, then turning and learning the next page and then the next page and then turning the pages and learning the pages and learning the next page and the next page.

And after a while of turning the pages they find they become more absorbed in the studying experience and less aware of the library around them. And like all good learning you need to take breaks and so they are aware that after studying for a while, they need to close the book, close their eyes and let their mind drift and daydream. Because people do, drift and daydream more frequently when they are studying and learning new things. Because it is your brains way of processing information. And so, after a while of studying that book they close the book, still allowing the music to play in their ears while they close their eyes and sit back in the chair for a moment and begin to go with the flow and let themselves drift and daydream.

And as they drift and daydream, so they find themselves imagining they are on a small little boat, gently rowing down a river, a very small river. And as they row down that river so they watch as a mother duck and a whole load of baby ducks swim down the river. And how those little baby ducklings bob around and get curious about things at the river bank. And then suddenly realise that because of curiosity, the other ducks have gone off ahead a little way and so they rush and kick their legs in a little rushy way to catch up with the other ducks to catch up a little bit, to try to push through the water a little faster to catch up with the group. And after a while another little duckling will become curious with something and the same thing happens again, that the little ducklings become curious and the mother duck has to keep looking back and keeping an eye on all those little ducks. And then the student just watches while gently rowing down the river as the mother duck jumps up onto the shore and then she sits there and turns and watches as the first of the little ducklings jumps up at the shore and plops back in the water and has to jump a few times flapping its little wings to get a foot-hold to make it up the bank and then the next duckling and the next duckling and the next, until there is just one left.

And the student watches as that one left struggles to get up that bank and the mother and all the other ducklings watch with expectant anticipation, as the duckling jumps up at the bank flapping its little wings and then jumps up again and again but keeps sliding down and then has to look and analyse and try and work out a different route. It is a little bit smaller than the others and so can't quite jump as high. So, it takes a look and works out a different route and then jumps up and finally manages to make it up onto the bank. Then the mother duck stands up and all of the ducklings and the mother walk off with the mother in front and all the ducklings following in a line behind her. And as she weaves and moves around different tufts of grass on the river bank, so the ducklings weave and move around those tufts as well. And the student continues rowing down the river.

And while continuing rowing down the river the student notices on the other bank, a beautiful little tabby cat and just watches as that cat seems to be walking around, doing its rounds of its territory, just checking everything is okay. It seems to be so relaxed, just walking gently around its territory. And the student watches that cat for a little while and then the cat stops and sits down looking graceful, sitting tall and just watches as the student rows by and the student watches back. And as the student continues to row, so they notice how the sky is beginning to turn a beautiful orange as the sun gently sets and while the sun is gently setting so the student can hear the sound of the oars in the water, sloshing of the river water against the bank, sounds of birds in the sky and the sounds of animals beginning to settle down for the night and so the student pulls the boat in to the shore, ties the boat to the shore and sets up a little tent on the shore of the river. And the student makes a small little campfire and cooks themselves some food while the fire crackles and pops and the light dances as the orange light of the sun lowers over the horizon and the blueness of the night starts to set in and the sounds of crickets and the evening and night-time animals start to appear and the breeze starts to cool down comfortably.

And the student eats some food and then sits there just gazing at the fire, listening to the surroundings as that fire burns down to embers, to a comfortable glow, letting off some warmth and while the student rests there, they become more tired and relaxed and the more tired and relaxed they become, the more they think about drifting off asleep, until eventually they lie back in the tent, they can hear the way the wind is blowing on the tent, moving the tent very slightly and gently in that wind, almost like it is lulling them to sleep, as they drift, comfortably asleep.

And while they drift comfortably asleep, so they begin to dream. They dream about walking along a hilltop overlooking the sea with their partner, holding hands, taking in the view, feeling the love of their partner and the love for their partner and then finding a bench, sitting on that bench, putting an arm around each other and gazing out over the ocean. And starting to wonder about the future, about hope, about what the future holds, the things they have got to look forward to, the type of things they can create for their future, plans that they have. And just then, someone walks past them and stops and says to them, did they know that there is a book that can give them tremendous insight, that can teach them about wisdom and life and what is important in life and what is not important in life and where priorities should lie. And they were curious about this. And the person said "All you have to do, is find the old lighthouse and you will find that book.".

And so together they got up, they decided to go to the lighthouse which was just a little way along from where they were. And they went all the way to that lighthouse. And the lighthouse was an unmanned lighthouse and they went into the lighthouse and they started exploring, they climbed up all the spiral stairs, checking different rooms. They went all the way up to the light, they then climbed all the way back down those spiral stairs having not found this book. They left the lighthouse and wondered where this book might be and what this book is. And then while exploring and discussing they learned that there used to be an old lighthouse and the old lighthouse used to be closer to the sea, but as the sea has come in, so they have had to move the lighthouse back and build a new one. So, they looked from the top of the hill to try and see evidence of an old lighthouse. And they could see where the old lighthouse must have been. They could see slightly out to sea that the way the water was flowing, something underneath the sea, something under the surface was disrupting the waves as they flowed by. So, they figured that must be where the old lighthouse was. They went down the hill, all the way down to the seashore, they got into a small boat and rowed out to where the water appeared to be separating and having the waves disrupted. Then the student got into the water, took a deep breath and dived down and he didn't have to go too far under the water to see that there was the ruins of an old lighthouse.

He dived down to the sea floor, swam into the ruins and saw a chest and he grabbed hold of the chest and swam back to the surface. And the student and their partner got that chest into their boat and rowed back to the shore. On the shore they placed the chest down, figured out how to open the chest, opened it and found this strange looking book. And they turned the page and then the next page and then the next page and every single page just had a mirror on it. And they didn't understand and they just turned all the pages all the way to the end of the book and every page just had a mirror on it. And they passed the book between each other, taking it in turns to look at the book, to look at different pages, to look at the back, to look at the front, to put it upside down, round the right way, back to front, front to back, whatever they did, they couldn't make sense of it.

And so, they just put it down on the sand between them and both sat, staring at the book in silence, working in their minds, trying to figure out, this book and the meaning of this book. And then, almost at exactly the same time, as if they were somehow synchronised, they looked at each other and could tell that the other one had worked out the meaning of the book. They smiled and opened the book. They smiled at the different pages. And then the student found himself waking up in the morning in the tent on the bank of the river to the sounds of morning birds, the smooth, running water sound of the river. He got back in his boat, having packed everything away and started rowing back the way he came. While he rowed back the way he came, he gradually found himself drifting back in his mind, starting to hear that music again and then noticing himself studying in the library, as he opened the book and carried on with his studying, looking forward to getting home later where he could drift and relax, comfortably asleep. Dreaming about that book, his experience and making sense of it all, because he was aware that it was a profound experience to learn from.

CONNECTING WITH NATURE

Steps for increasing effectiveness of the story:

1. What do you want to achieve from reading this?

2. Think about one thing you have achieved today.

3. Say to yourself "When I read this story then…"

Alternative introduction:

"As I read this and begin to drift comfortably asleep, I don't know whether I will find myself drifting asleep more to the sound of my voice or the words I read, or perhaps to the spaces between the words. And as I drift comfortably asleep I'll just read this story to myself."

Connecting with Nature

As you listen to me and begin to drift comfortably asleep, you can make sure you are comfortable and you can close your eyes and I don't know whether you will drift more comfortably asleep with the sound of my voice, with the spaces between my words, or with the words themselves. And so, as you drift comfortably asleep, you can listen to me tell this story in the background.

And there was a lady who enjoyed going out camping, she enjoyed her own company, she enjoyed peace and solitude, she enjoyed being one with nature and felt that being one with nature and being out camping on your own helped to connect with the world around you. Helped to keep you grounded. And so, she decided to go out camping and with her backpack on her back she trekked out into the countryside, trekked through woodland, enjoying the sounds of the birds, hearing a woodpecker at a tree, the sound of a distant stream, the sounds of rustling leaves as the wind blows a breeze. The sound of each footstep, the smells in the woods and occasionally she would touch a branch of a tree to feel that connection, to feel the sensations of the bark on her fingertips. She would stop and watch butterflies dancing around flowers and the way beams of light would dance through the canopies above. And she appreciated the reduced sound that you get in the woods, the way everything just seems so much more peaceful and calm.

And after some time, walking through the woods, she found herself reaching a gate, passing through that gate and entering into a vast meadow with hills either side, deer off in the distance, just grazing and watching out. She could see birds flying overhead and other animals in the meadow and all the different wild flowers. And she set up a camp, up on the hillside, overlooking the meadow. Able to look one way to the woodland, able to look the other way further down into the meadow, all the way down to the lake way off in the distance. And she prepared her area and created a campfire and set up a tent and then sat down just inside that tent in front of the campfire, listening to the crackling fire as the fire began to burn down until it was just giving off heat, no flames, just glowing embers by nightfall. And as the sun set, so she began to hear and notice bats flying overhead catching insects and just the calming sounds of the outdoors. And she could feel the warmth of the fire as she sat just inside her tent having something to eat. And she enjoyed this experience, she valued this experience, of being able to look up and see the stars across the sky, of noticing the way the firelight makes shadows dance and seems almost hypnotic as you gaze at it.

And as she sat there gazing at the fire she started eating an apple, enjoying the sweetness of the apple. Valuing the way that the apple was created with its skin to hold the goodness in. And then she noticed that it was starting to rain a bit. And she had camped in all conditions and she liked it when it rained. She felt it calming and comforting. So, she backed into her tent, climbed into her sleeping bag, zipped up the entrance to the tent, she knew her tent was well and truly grounded, safe and secure. And at first, she could hear large drops of water hitting the fabric of the tent and she had a light on inside the tent, just hanging above her and she could notice the drops of rain hitting the tent and those drops started large and infrequent and gradually started to get more frequent as the rain got heavier outside. And she knew that the rain would put the fire out and as she was approaching bedtime anyway she wasn't going to need the fire. She was plenty warm enough in her sleeping bag in her tent. And she just rested back in that sleeping back, felt all snuggly, warm and cosy. Just listening to the way the rain bounced on the tent. The way the wind made the sides of the tent move and she found it so calming, so relaxing. A bit like sitting in a conservatory on a rainy day or sitting in a car on a rainy day. Just being able to listen to that rain while keeping dry and warm and comfortable.

And she relaxed back listening to the rain and found that the rain was rhythmically guiding her asleep. And although she was attempting to keep her attention focused on the rain, on enjoying the sound of the rain, her eyes would flicker and she would find that she kept dropping off asleep for a moment at a time, until she totally fell asleep deeply and comfortably. And the next thing she knew, she woke up in the morning feeling so refreshed and revitalised, to the sounds of birds and morning animals announcing the morning. She opened the tent and saw the sunlight and breathed in the fresh air that seemed even more fresh, as if the rain had washed any pollutants out of the air. She could see the morning dew across the meadow, across the plants, see some of it turning to mist as the sun continued to rise. And she climbed out of the tent, stretched herself and then went and prepared herself for the morning, restarted the fire, to make herself some breakfast and a cup of tea, boiled a pot of water and just loved that moment when the pot would start whistling to let her know that she is ready to poor the tea and that feeling of drinking a tea in the countryside out of a flask cup or a camping cup, rather than a typical mug at home. Something about holding that cup in her hands, feeling the warmth of that tea.

And she just sat back and enjoyed the view, enjoyed looking down towards the lake, enjoyed looking over to the woodland, enjoyed watching the birds in the sky. And she knew the grass was still slightly damp from the night before, but if it wasn't for that, you would almost not have realised that it had rained. Because of the fact that there were no clouds in the sky, everything was just blue in every direction. And the air was fresh and cool and she could feel it in her nostrils, feel it on her skin and she rested there, drinking a tea, enjoying a moments peace and solitude, enjoying this time inside her mind, with her own thoughts and ideas about nature, about what there is to enjoy in life, to look forward to in life, to appreciate in life. As she gazed down at the meadow and she thought it was curious how every single blade of grass is actually unique and different to every other single blade of grass, yet at a glance, you could just assume that all those blades of grass are just a blade of grass looking like any other blade of grass and it is only when you get down to each blade and truly and honestly take a close look at each blade of grass that you notice that each one is slightly different to each other one and yet all of that difference doesn't take away from the beauty of the meadow, the harmony of the meadow, the way everything seems connected, the way everything seems to have a purpose out here in the country and she enjoyed her little insights like this.

Like the sadness of a predator catching its prey and yet had the predator not caught the prey, it wouldn't have turned out so well for the predator or the predator's offspring. Or the joy when the prey gets away and how that turns out well for the prey's offspring. And how everything, from the blades of grass to the deer, to the birds of prey, how everything is connected in a balance. And she is just an observer on this. And she enjoyed having thoughts like this, thoughts that allowed her to connect, to understand deeper meaning and to have an appreciation for the world around her. She could almost feel the countryside in her heart, as if she was one, in-step, in rhythm, in harmony with the countryside, with the world around her. Able to just enjoy being in the moment. Not trapped in the past in her mind, worrying about other things, not trapped in the future in her mind, worrying about what might be, but enjoying being in the here and now, accepting that what is, is. And just enjoying what she can do here and now.

And during the day, as the sun grows higher, she kept her camp set up, she wandered away from her camp, she wandered down the hill, she wandered through the meadow down towards the lake, she walked all the way to the lake and barefooted she walked in to the lake, just a little way in, to feel the water, to feel the coolness of the water on her feet as it flowed and lapped gently on the shore. And gazed down through that water at small fish swimming around her feet, tickling her toes, darting out of the way whenever she moved her feet and then coming back again when her feet were stationary. And she just stood there with her eyes closed, breathing in and out, the fresh air, the way the air smelled even fresher over the water, enjoying the way the sun glistened on the lake, the way the breeze blew across the lake. Enjoyed the peace and silence here. With no-one else around, just her in nature. Able to connect, no worries, no phones, no distractions, just a connection with the environment.

And through the day she wandered around the lake, sat by the lake, meditated, took in the environment and felt a connection with the environment. She had something to eat at lunch time and then as it approached the end of the day she went back to her tent to settle down for another night. And again, she lit a fire, just for some light and a bit of warmth in the evening and to cook some food with. And she had something to eat in the evening, listened to the cracking fire, felt its warmth, enjoyed the way that shadows danced, the flames flickered, as that fire gradually burned down to just embers. And then when she was ready and felt it was time to sleep, she moved back into the tent, zipped up the entrance, laid down in her sleeping bag and just listened to the evening sounds outside. And as she listened to those evening sounds outside, so she began to breathe deep comfortable breaths, with each exhalation being longer than each inhalation, having a sense of a connection with the world around her, focusing on her breathing and other sounds around her, as she began to drift comfortably asleep and as she drifted comfortably asleep so she drifted into some comfortable dreams for the night and she knew she was going to enjoy those dreams, before waking in the morning feeling so calm and refreshed, to enjoy another day on this hillside and in this valley and she knew she was going to spend a few more days out here, exploring and enjoying being one with nature before deciding to take down her tents and head back to normality. But she was going to make the most of her time here first and she thought all that as she drifted comfortably, relaxed, asleep.

THE COUPLE'S 'FROZEN IN TIME' TRIP

Steps for increasing effectiveness of the story:

1. What do you want to achieve from reading this?

2. Think about one thing you have achieved today.

3. Say to yourself "When I read this story then…"

Alternative introduction:

"As I read this and begin to drift comfortably asleep, I don't know whether I will find myself drifting asleep more to the sound of my voice or the words I read, or perhaps to the spaces between the words. And as I drift comfortably asleep I'll just read this story to myself."

The Couple's 'Frozen in Time' Trip

As you take a moment to close your eyes and get yourself comfortable and begin to drift off to sleep, you can listen to me talking in the background and as you listen to me talking in the background, I don't know whether you will drift deeper asleep with the sound of my voice, with the words that I use, or whether you will drift deeper asleep faster with the spaces between my words. And as you comfortably drift off to sleep, I'm going to tell you a story about a couple who lived in a castle.

This couple enjoyed their life in the castle. They worked in the castle, they spent a lot of their time in the castle grounds, they occasionally ventured out to the nearby village and this couple felt that they had a very lucky life. One day they decided to go on a trip together, they wanted to go somewhere different, they decided to go away for a few days. They packed some bags and decided they were going to go camping, going to go off and just see where they end up. They left the castle, left the grounds and began to walk down towards the nearby village. They walked along that road towards the nearby village and as they walked they looked around them, they admired the countryside, they could see people working in fields, they could see birds flying above the nearby woodland, they noticed the colour of the sky, felt the warmth of the sun on their skin and could listen to the footsteps they were taking and how both of them had their footsteps fall in time with each other. They wandered into the village, walked through the village, wandered by the market stalls and bought themselves some food and a few other bits and pieces as they continued their journey through the village and then out the other side of the village. And they were walking down towards the nearby lake and then they were going to follow the lake along to a river and then they would follow the river and they had never gone much further than the lake before, so they didn't know where the path along the edge of the river would take them.

So, they walked through the village and continued walking down towards that lake and the lake was slightly down a hill and they chatted to each other as they walked, while they enjoyed the environment. They were both curious about what they would discover. And as they reached the lake, they decided to stop for a bite to eat, they laid down a mat on the ground, they sat on the mat and they ate some food and they rested back and they enjoyed some of the sun, relaxing sound of the water lashing on the shore, just enjoyed having a comfortable experience. And then later in the afternoon they decided to continue their journey. They continued around the lake, around to the river. And started following the river. And after a few hours they noticed how the sun was beginning to set and they were approaching some woodland and they were already beyond where they normally walked in this direction. So, they took some time, to set up camp and have a rest. They made a little fire, they set up a tent and they settled down for the night, enjoying this adventure together. And as the sun set and the moon rose, so the stars brightened the sky, as they drifted comfortably asleep.

In the morning they felt awake and alert to continue their journey. After some time, the path along the edge of the river seemed to come to an end. They didn't know which way to go, so they decided to walk off road, to cut through the woods. They cut through the woods, went off road. And after a while, they discovered an unusual looking tree. They walked up and touched that tree. They ran their fingers around the bark and they noticed that this tree was artificial. And that the tree was against a steep cliff and it almost looked like it was built into the cliff, that somehow this tree, if it wasn't artificial had grown partially in the cliff, but they could tell there was something different about this. It looked like a tree, it felt like a tree, but they could tell it was artificial. And as they were running their fingers around the bark, feeling what this tree felt like, suddenly a door opened in the tree and they decided that they were trying to have an adventure, so they would walk through that door. So, they walked through the door into that tree and it was a path, which led them into this cliff.

So, they followed this path and they walked into the cliff and they closed the door behind them, lit a torch and walked into the cliff. The sounds changed as they walked inside this cliff. The feeling of the air changed while they were inside the cliff. And they followed this secret path, unsure where it would take them. And after some time of walking, along this secret path, they found a chamber deep inside this cliff. In this chamber was a glowing blue pool of water in the centre and they walked over to that glowing pool of water and they put their hands in, to feel the water and it felt warm and comfortable. And then they sat there and they lowered their legs in and it felt refreshing. And while they sat there with their legs dangling in the water, so they noticed some of that glowing passing up and over them. And it felt so comfortable, so comforting and calming. Then that light engulfed them and it was almost like the light and the water were the same thing, almost like the water had covered their whole body, a little bit like sweat, only without a sweaty feeling.

They climbed out of the water, tried to dry themselves off but found that this glowing continued to remain on them. They didn't worry, it felt comfortable, but they wondered what it was. They saw a door at the back of this chamber. They opened the door and realised they were high up in a cliff with a path leading down into a valley full of trees. And as they looked out, suddenly they realised that at first glance they hadn't noticed, but the birds flying in formation over the valley hadn't moved. Initially they didn't pay attention to this, but on reflection they realised those birds were stationary. They noticed there was a stillness to the air and they walked themselves down the path from that point in the cliff and they walked their way down into the valley and they couldn't hear any sounds of the leaves rustling, they couldn't hear any sounds of birds singing. They couldn't hear the sounds of their own footsteps.

They realised, somehow, everything had frozen. They didn't know how. They wondered whether time had stopped, or whether they had come out of time in some way because of that water. They walked along the valley exploring as they went. They saw different animals not moving anywhere. Some animals were 'mid-whatever' they were doing. There was a squirrel hovering in the air, mid-jump from tree to tree and there were birds hovering motionless in the air. They explored with curiosity. They didn't know, or understand what was going on, but they knew this was a curious experience.

As they walked through the valley they found a clearing. They walked out into the clearing and could see stationary insects over certain plants. And they continued walking and they settled down to have a picnic and found something unusual about this environment, that it was weird being out in nature like this and yet having no sounds at all. And they found that a really weird experience and they also found it a beautiful experience and they enjoyed their picnic. And they noticed that the light or the water was dissipating from their bodies, in the same way that you just dry out in the sun over time. And as it was dissipating, so time appeared to be moving very slowly and the more they dried off in the sun, the faster time appeared to go until after quite a while, suddenly time seemed to be going at normal speed again, they could hear the breeze again, they could notice rustling of leave in the trees, see the movement of plants, insects flying around, birds flying around. And they thought it was a curious experience.

And they knew they were supposed to learn something from the experience and they had wondered what they would learn. And they felt like they had a sense of wonder and serenity, it was a certain serene feeling regarding the experience they had. They discussed with each other, the importance of being in the moment. Of making the most of each moment, rather than being in the future, worrying about what the future might hold, or worrying about what might happen in the future, or being in the past and worrying about what has happened in the past, or worrying what people might think, but just being in the moment. And they felt that was perhaps what was being taught to them, to learn to be in the moment and be able to appreciate what is here and now. And they enjoyed their food and then the sun was setting again and so they sat down in the valley, they set up camp, sat out talking most of the night with a campfire, enjoying the cracking of the campfire. Watching how the shadows danced with each flickering flame and the smell of that campfire, before relaxing down for the night, gazing up at the stars, watching them twinkle and dance, wondering if there is anyone out there on a planet somewhere, lying down gazing up at the stars, watching them twinkle up in the night sky for them, wondering if there is anyone out there looking back at them. And they put an arm around each other and held each other tight and drifted comfortably asleep.

The next morning they awoke, ate breakfast and they took in the environment, they were aware this was the last chance to see this environment for a while and they walked back, up to the cave and they walked through the cave and they came out of that door in that fake tree. Walked through the woods and found their way back to the river. They camped again another night by the river before following that river all the way back to the lake and they felt themselves walking slower, trying to make this trip last slightly longer, really trying to take in and absorb the experience, enjoy the experience, enjoy the companionship, enjoy the company of each other, enjoy making the most of this time together.

And they looked out over the lake and they saw people fishing, they saw people on boats, they admired the way the water flowed, the way the ripples moved, the way the air smelled fresh as it blew off the lake. They worked their way back up towards the village and they stopped at the village to talk to friends about the trip they had been on, they didn't say where that tree was exactly, but they talked about the trip they had been on, about some of the things they had seen, some of the things they had learned. Then they headed back to the castle, to the familiar surroundings of their home, their workplace.

And they settled down for the night, knowing that they had work in the morning. They settled down for the night, still talking to each other about their time away, about the experience they had just had, about the last few days exploring and how they looked forward to going exploring again in the future and whether they would go the same way and do the same kind of thing, or go a different way and learn something new and find something else out. And they started already planning their future, planning future trips and gradually their conversations calmed down as they found themselves gently and relaxing, drifting off to sleep in each other's arms, so calmly and relaxed, asleep.

DADDY AND DAUGHTER'S FISHING TRIP

Steps for increasing effectiveness of the story:

1. What do you want to achieve from reading this?
2. Think about one thing you have achieved today.
3. Say to yourself "When I read this story then…"

Alternative introduction:

"As I read this and begin to drift comfortably asleep, I don't know whether I will find myself drifting asleep more to the sound of my voice or the words I read, or perhaps to the spaces between the words. And as I drift comfortably asleep I'll just read this story to myself."

So, as you begin to drift comfortably asleep, I don't know whether you will find yourself drifting to sleep faster with the sound of my voice, with the words that I am using, or whether it will be with the spaces between my words.

And as you comfortably begin to drift off to sleep, I will tell you a story in the background, a story of a young girl who keeps wanting to spend some time with her dad, but her dad is always busy, her dad is always working or wanting to relax and have time for himself.

Every day the girl asks;

"Will you spend time with me today?"

And every day he is always too busy. Eventually just as she is giving up hope and yet still keeps trying, he responds by saying he wants to take her fishing, he wants to teach her how to fish. The girl didn't really have an interest in fishing, but was interested in spending time with her father, so the two of them, the next morning, woke up, packed for the fishing trip and set off to a nearby lake. As they arrived at the lake, so the girl looked around. She enjoyed the smell of that fresh air, the breeze on her face, there were a few clouds in the sky. She could see trees around the edge of the lake and lush grass. No-one else seemed to be around. Her father said took her down to a boat.

He carried a lot of the fishing gear as she carried a little. They got on the boat. The father started to row out into the middle of the lake and then the daughter asked if she could have a go at rowing and so she rowed that boat towards the middle of the lake. At first, she struggled to get the coordination between the left and the right oar and they kept going around in circles and then weaving the other way and then the other way and sometimes the oar wouldn't go into the water right and it would splash water up into her father's face and he was laughing with her and she was laughing at him.

And they rowed out into the middle of the lake, pulled the oars onto the boat and just allowed the boat to bob up and down in the middle of the lake. The father then baited the fishing hook and demonstrated how to get that hook as far away from the boat as possible into the water. And he whipped that rod as the reel un-spun and the hook shot off and plopped into the water. She then got her smaller fishing rod and facing the opposite side of the boat, she copied her dad and whipped the rod and almost straightaway got it right by copying him. And the hook plopped into the water. And he said

"You just have to sit and wait, just sit silently and patiently and feel the rod, feel any subtle movement, sensations. What you are looking for is a sign that a fish has bitten on the bait and a slight tug on that hook and that slight tug with translate into a slight movement at the tip of the rod which will be felt at the handle and you just have to be able to sit and wait and focus on the feelings, focus on the sensations. It's about becoming in tune with those feelings and sensations, learning to notice the most subtle response and to be able to begin to learn the difference between a lifeless piece of weed catching on that hook and a fish and you can begin to learn the different way both feel, the different way different things feel, through your fingertips, through the palms of your hands holding onto that rod, so that you will know when to reel that fish in. And when reeling a fish in, it is about sensitivity, reel too fast and you will lose the fish, reel too slow and you will lose the fish, so you have to reel at just the right speed, which requires sensitivity to know when to reel faster or slower and when to pause reeling in or reeling out and it is almost like falling into a dance with the fish on the end of that line. And so it is with many other things in life, all you have to do is learn to transfer skills from one area to another. There are people you need to deal with in life, like fish and situations you need to deal with like this and so fishing will teach more about life than just how to fish."

The girl had a sense that she kind of understood, but she didn't know how you transfer skills from one part of life to another, but she trusted that somehow it must happen and she was enjoying her fishing trip with her father. It was these kinds of experiences that she wanted, something where she learned from the wisdom of her dad. After a few hours of fishing on that lake, her father had caught a few fish and yet nothing had bitten her line. And she was wondering whether she was doing something wrong. So, the father taught her a trick, a way of wiggling the rod, of pulling the line in and out a little bit to create movement at the hook, which creates curiosity and intrigue. She did this and suddenly she got a bite and excitedly she started reeling in this fish, following her father's instructions, not too fast, not too slow, sometimes letting the line go, sometimes pulling the line in, pulling on the rod and loosening the rod and eventually she got the fish to the boat. She had a photo taken with that fish before she unhooked it and threw it back and then she decided it was starting to get a bit late and she was starting to get hungry. It was just after lunch time and she had been there for hours, so the father suggested, why don't they row down the river, as he knows this nice place to stop.

The father and his daughter set off across the lake to the river and started rowing down the river. They rowed past people walking on the bank and she loved just sitting back, closing her eyes and feeling the warmth of the sun and the breeze on her face, as they rowed, as she listened to the sound of the oars, as they pushed the water behind them while she would occasionally talk to her father and he would talk back and she had this strong feeling that she was creating something beautiful in her mind which will last with her forever. And as they carried on rowing, they saw dog walkers on the shore, some people just sitting there eating sandwiches, some people waved and said hello, for no reason at all other than that they were passing by and after a little while they arrived at a little pier area, somewhere to dock up the boat and so the father navigated the boat alongside the pier, tied the boat to the side, helped his daughter off and then climbed off the boat himself.

They were at a beautiful country hotel. They walked up to the hotel and were going to the restaurant of this hotel. They sat outside overlooking the river. The father went in to the hotel, got some menus and returned, they looked at the menus and decided what they would like to eat. Someone came outside and served them, they ordered a couple of drinks and ordered their food and they sat just peacefully with the mumble of voices in the background, just sat and enjoyed the view, enjoyed gazing over the river, watching others in boats of different kinds occasionally pass by, enjoying some relaxing time with dad and daughter.

Then their food came out, they ate their food and had a little talk with each other about their interests, mainly the dad asking what the daughter liked to do, asking what was going on in her life at the moment. While her mouth was answering her mind was thinking about the fact that he was totally focused on her, he wasn't thinking about work, thinking about other things, thinking about what time he had to go, he appeared totally interested in her and what she had to say and totally in that moment with her and she felt so loved and valued and respected in that moment and knew that her father being like this, was teaching her more than just giving her a nice experience as a dad. Teaching her about the way people interact and communicate meaningfully with each other and after eating, they had another drink and continued sitting there and she realised it was now getting well into the afternoon and the sun was beginning to set. The sky was starting to turn the most beautiful orange.

They left the hotel and went and sat on the pier with their feet dangling over the edge, just continuing talking as the sun started getting lower over the horizon and then before the sun had fully set the dad said it was time to start heading back home. To head down the river, back to that lake and back to the shore before it gets too dark.

And as the sun was beginning its journey over the horizon they got back in the boat and the dad rowed the boat back along the river towards the lake and the daughter continued to savour this moment, to savour this day. And then they arrived at the lake, the moon was more visible in the sky now, starting to shine brightly. The sun was almost totally set, it had long gone over the horizon, but there was enough light still to just about make out the shore, so the dad rowed to the shore and he said to his daughter "do you want to know how to start a fire? And do you want an experience of camping, just for a few hours, to really make the end of this day special?" He thought this would round off the day. Obviously when they get home they will go to bed, but for now she could have this experience and he could teach her about camping.

The daughter wanted this experience, so together they gathered up some wood from among the nearby trees, he demonstrated clearing an area to make sure the fire wouldn't set fire to anything it isn't supposed to, he demonstrated stacking the wood and making it so that it would light and then he lit the fire and the daughter got two chairs out of the car, set up those chairs near the fire. The dad got some food out of an ice box and they cooked up that food and enjoyed watching the last of the sunlight, watching how the stars appeared more in the sky twinkling above, the way the moonlight now glistened on the lake and then after a little while the dad said it was time for them to go home, so they put out the fire, packed everything away and made their journey back home. And on the journey home the daughter and the dad continued talking and bonding and the daughter said she wanted to do this kind of thing more often, she didn't want it to be just a one-off.

The dad said he needed to make more effort, he said he could get so wrapped up in work, in what he feels he needs to do, so that he forgets to focus on what he should do and sometimes life can pass you by while you are busy focusing on something else and when there are loved ones involved you don't want that to be the case and he told her the trip had taught him a lot about where his priorities should be and how he should focus his attention. And the daughter closed her eyes and just listened as the car drove along, just listened to the sounds around them, with a smile on her face, reminiscing about the day she has just had and hoping that this is the first of many. On arriving home, she kissed her dad, went up to bed, got into bed and allowed herself to drift into a pleasant dream as she began to drift off comfortably asleep.

DOWN THE PREHISTORIC RABBIT HOLE

Steps for increasing effectiveness of the story:

1. What do you want to achieve from reading this?

2. Think about one thing you have achieved today.

3. Say to yourself "When I read this story then…"

Alternative introduction:

"As I read this and begin to drift comfortably asleep, I don't know whether I will find myself drifting asleep more to the sound of my voice or the words I read, or perhaps to the spaces between the words. And as I drift comfortably asleep I'll just read this story to myself."

As you comfortably begin to drift off to sleep, I don't know whether you will drift deeper with the sound of my voice, or whether it will be with the spaces between my words, or whether it will be that you drift deeper and more comfortably asleep with the words that I use. And so, as you drift comfortably asleep, I'm just going to tell you a story in the background. And while I tell that story you can fall asleep comfortably.

There was a girl out in her garden one day. She was playing and running around and then she had the most unusual experience, while she was playing she saw a rabbit hole. It was an unusually large rabbit hole, so she went over to that hole and peered inside. It was dark, so she decided to crawl inside a little bit to get a better look. As she crawled in she noticed the hole got larger and larger, until eventually the hole was large enough for her to stand up and walk in. And as she walked along the inside of this rabbit hole, so she noticed that it turned from having mud all around the sides, to merging into having concrete or some other manmade materials all around the sides, which gradually merged into looking like a corridor, with flat sides, a flat roof, an echoey concrete floor and a glow at the end of this corridor which continued to get brighter as she walked closer to it with curiosity. She reached out with her hand and ran her fingers over the wall, curious about the way the wall seemed to turn from mud into concrete. She was aware of the way her footsteps were now echoing down the corridor and she could look back and see that rabbit hole and yet when she looked forward, it looked like there was a glow at a door, or something off in the distance.

And with a sense of calm curiosity she walked her way towards that door and when she arrived at that door she saw that it looked like a lift, she pressed the button next to the door and waited and waited and she could hear movement behind the door, the sound of a lift descending and she waited and waited and then with a ping, the door slid open and she walked inside the lift. And she thought that this was a very peculiar situation, a very strange thing to happen, she saw that there were five levels and decided that she would just go all the way to the bottom and so she pressed one.

She waited a moment as the door slid shut and the lift began to lower, from five, to four, to three and she could see light passing by the lift as the movement continued to happen, to two, to one, where the lift stopped and the door slid open. She walked out of the lift and found herself in a vast cavern, as if somehow this lift had taken her down into a cave. She wondered whether this cave was underneath her back garden, because she didn't know anything about this. She started exploring. Walking around the outside of the cave initially, touching the cave wall, getting a feel for it, hearing the occasional drip of water echoing through the cave, hearing the way her footsteps echoed around the cave. She couldn't hear any other noises in the cave. After a while, she saw something that looked a bit different in the cave wall. Something that looked like it was artificial but made to blend in, made to look like part of the cave.

She pushed against this artificial area and pulled on it and felt around it, trying to find any clue. Eventually she knocked into a stone on the floor and realised that although it looked like it was a stone that should have moved, just like a loose stone or pebble, it didn't go anywhere, so she kicked it again and noticed it still didn't go anywhere. She lent down, felt around on that stone and realised that it was like a lever that could be pulled upwards. She pulled that stone upwards, let go and it popped back down into place. And as it did, the wall beside her slid backwards and disappeared, opening up a secret tunnel. And she walked into this secret tunnel, feeling curiouser and curiouser the deeper she went into the experience and the weirdest thing happened, as she was approaching the end of the tunnel, so everything started to get lighter as if she was walking towards daylight. And she continued walking and she started hearing the sounds of birds and the sounds of other animals she didn't recognise. And she could feel a breeze on her face and she exited the tunnel and realised she was partway up a cliff overlooking a vast valley with trees and grasses and above looked like a sky with clouds and yet she was aware that she was inside the ground and this must be a huge cave and she couldn't understand how the ceiling here is glowing like normal daylight. She couldn't see where the sun was, but it looked as normal as when she is outside in the woods normally.

She saw that there was a path down to the bottom of the valley and she followed that path and she could feel the breeze on her face. She could smell the woodland smell, smell the wood and plants, hear the animals. Then as she looked around in the valley, she noticed something she didn't initially believe and had to double check. It looked like there were dinosaurs in this valley. There were pterodactyls in the sky and it was like a prehistoric world and some of the plants had vast flat leaves, others looked like unusual conifers. And apart from grasses, there didn't seem to be very many flowers that she could see. She was fascinated by this; somehow, she had found her way to a prehistoric world and she started exploring in this prehistoric world, climbing up a tree, watching as giant dinosaurs walked past. Really getting absorbed in this prehistoric world.

Then she noticed, off in the distance, by a lake, it looked like there was a person there. So, she decided she wanted to go and talk with them and find out what this place is. She climbed down from the tree and carefully worked her way through the valley, she had this feeling like everything was perfectly fine and safe, but she wanted to be careful nonetheless. So, she walked down the valley, breathing in the smells, feeling the grass and the air on her face, noticing the sound of each footstep. And as she continued down the valley, she could see the person was just milling around, doing something at the lake and she got closer and closer and noticed that they looked like they were a scientist and eventually she managed to get to where they were. And she kept just out of sight and watched them working and they were testing the water and taking a sample and they were testing the air and writing down some notes. They were taking a few pictures and they were wheeling something and they put their samples on the thing they were wheeling and they started heading around the outside of the lake. The girl carefully and quietly followed and watched as they reached the cabin and went in to the cabin and she wondered whether she should follow, whether she should knock on the cabin door and introduce herself.

After a little while she decided that is what she would do, she had to know what this place was, she had her curiosity and she wanted to know and so she knocked on the door and she could see through the window that the person appeared startled, but they came to the door and they saw the girl stood there. They asked who she was, how she had found them and why she was here? She said "Those were the questions I was going to ask you. Who are you? Why are you here? Where is here?"

The person invited her in. She sat down in that cabin and could feel a certain coolness and comfort inside the cabin. She asked him, "Where is here and who are you?"

And they wanted to know the same from her. They explained that they created this place, they have spent their life creating this place. They have had a fascination with the prehistoric world, with saving things and they had managed years earlier to create this prehistoric world underground and they are the master of this world. Their role is to watch over it, to do as little as possible without interfering with it, but just monitor it and make sure it ticks along okay.

And the girl found this interesting. She said that she had got there by following a rabbit hole and the master realised that somehow, maybe a rabbit, maybe a different animal had obviously burrowed into the ground and had somehow managed to burrow into one of the corridors of this base, this underground facility. So, this curious girl had followed that into this underground facility and she had so many questions about it, about how it was made, about the size of it, about how they have recreated the sun. How they make sure there is enough oxygen and the correct composition of the air and that the plants can grow and where they got all of these prehistoric plants and animals. The scientist explained everything, they normally didn't talk to anyone, so they enjoyed having someone who was interested in all of this who they could talk to about it all. They talked about how this was a secret place that no-one was to know about. The girl swore that she would also keep it secret. They said, this is somewhere they find a sense of wonder and serenity, a sense of peace, a sense of being back to a time before lots of chaos. To a simpler time. They explained about how they enjoy relaxing by the lake, just doing their job, gathering some samples, feeding that information back, relaxing in the cabin. Watching dinosaurs, pterodactyls and other animals going about their lives. Just as they would have done millions and millions of years earlier.

They find that this is their safe place, this is their place away from the hustle and bustle of the 'real world' and when they go home they have to hear cars and traffic and have lots of chaos and yet here they can enjoy peace and serenity and have a sense of wonder. The girl appreciated all of this. But, she also realised that she was away from home and as far as anyone thought, she was playing in the garden, but now she has played far out of the garden. So, she left the cabin, she was told that if she kept it a secret she could come and visit again. She left the cabin, wandered back through the valley, climbed up to that secret tunnel, she followed that secret tunnel and found her way back to the lift. And then back to the corridor and then eventually back to her garden. She sat down in her garden, relaxing under a tree, thinking about the experience she had just had and while she relaxed there thinking about the experience she had just had, her mind drifted and dreamed and floated off as she comfortably and relaxed, fell asleep.

FALLING ASLEEP IN A RAINFOREST

Steps for increasing effectiveness of the story:

1. What do you want to achieve from reading this?

2. Think about one thing you have achieved today.

3. Say to yourself "When I read this story then…"

Alternative introduction:

"As I read this and begin to drift comfortably asleep, I don't know whether I will find myself drifting asleep more to the sound of my voice or the words I read, or perhaps to the spaces between the words. And as I drift comfortably asleep I'll just read this story to myself."

As you listen to me and begin to fall asleep, I'm going to tell you a story in the background. And as you drift comfortably asleep, you can have a sense of somebody who was going about everyday life, waking up, going through their life, going to work, being polite to others, going home, watching some TV going to bed, getting up, going to work, being polite to others, going home and watching some TV and going to bed. And every day this was their routine. They would wake up, go to work, go home, watch TV and go to bed. Then one day, they woke up and they thought to themselves that they didn't want to keep doing this. They wished that there was something more exciting in life, because when they were thinking back over their past, only a few memories stood out. Most of the memories just blurred into one. They couldn't tell one day from the next, just getting up, going to work, going home, watching TV and going to bed.

One day while they were at home, they decided to take a look on the internet and randomly book a holiday. A trip anywhere at all, they didn't know where, they just wanted to book something. They booked a holiday to an exotic location and all of a sudden while they were going to work they found themselves thinking about the excitement of the trip away that they have coming up in the future. While they were at work working and smiling politely they were, in their mind thinking about what this exotic location would be like. On their journey home they were thinking about that holiday they were going to be going on and looking forward to it. And every day they crossed off a date on the diary as they got closer and closer to their trip. And then the holiday came around and they travelled to that exotic location, the plane landed, they went to the hotel and left their stuff in the hotel. They decided to go out exploring. They went out exploring and wandered out into a beautiful rainforest. Listening to the sounds of the birds, the rustling of the leaves, the sounds of monkeys in the distance and all of the other sounds.

They could feel how warm it was in the rainforest. Their attention was so focused on the excitement on the exploration. They could hear water in the distance and so they pushed through the rainforest. The sound of the water got louder and louder and they continued pushing through the rainforest excited, wondering what they would find. The sound of the water continued to get louder and louder until eventually they found a clearing. Suddenly there was the light from the sun beating down on them, that glistened on the water of the giant lake surrounded by huge waterfalls. They could see huge waterfalls and the spray and mist coming up from the bottom of the waterfalls and rainbows dancing in the spray above the lake. They saw what looked like a small wooden boat down on the lake, they walked down to the boat, climbed into the boat, picked up the oars, pushed off the side and gently paddled out into the lake. They could feel the force of the water against the oars as they paddled. They paddled out towards the centre of the lake. The lake was calm here in the centre, the water quickly calming as it moved away from the waterfalls. The lake appeared to be deep. The person pulled the oars into the boat, put their backpack down to use as a pillow, laid back in the boat, closed their eyes and relaxed listening to the waterfalls in the background, smelling the fresh water air. Feeling the subtlest rocking of the boat on the lake and feeling the warmth of the sun beating down on them.

With their eyes closed, they took some deep breaths and relaxed. They allowed themselves to become absorbed in the moment. And as they relaxed and became absorbed in the moment, the sun continued its journey across the sky, gradually lowering in the sky and the sounds in the forest began to change, from daytime sounds to night time sounds. And as the sun set, so the person opened their eyes and gazed up into the sky. And as they gazed up into the sky, they could see the blanket of stars twinkling, different colours in the sky, different clouds. And they could see the Milky Way stretching across the sky. They recognised one point of light in the sky as being Mars. And as they gazed at that point of light, as they gazed up at Mars, so their eyes began to close again. And as their eyes began to close, they discovered their eyes opening actually *on* the red planet. And oddly they didn't have any space gear on and they were able to breathe perfectly fine, as if they were just on Earth, but they know they were on the red planet.

And they discovered themselves at the foot of a mountain range on Mars. And they thought "Wouldn't it be exciting to climb a mountain range on Mars?" And so, they climbed the mountain, they trekked up the mountain. And as they approached the summit they noticed how vibrant the colour red was. They began to get a new perspective on this world. They sat down and they enjoyed the view, knowing they were the first person ever to step foot here. And as the small sun set on Mars, so they could see two small moons in the sky and all of the stars in the sky and they could see off in the distance, a pale blue dot and they knew it was Earth. And they enjoyed the awe, the wonder of gazing at that pale blue dot. Knowing all life on Earth, all known life in the universe, is on that pale blue dot. Suddenly they had a sense that life seems so fragile when it is all contained in that one location and such a small location from this distance. They felt a sense of love and compassion for all that life. And a sense of the importance of looking after that pale blue dot. And as the sun rose on another Martian day, with these new learnings they climbed down the mountain. And as they reached the base of the mountain, so they found their eyes opening in the boat floating on the lake, listening to that water, feeling the warmth of the morning sun.

They got the oars and rowed back to shore. They continued exploring for a while in the rainforest before deciding to pitch up a tent to camp in the rainforest. They pitched the tent up tied between the trees, positioned a few feet off the ground where you can climb up into the tent and be a few feet off the ground. In the tent, you feel like you are floating. And as they relaxed in the tent, feeling comfortable and calm, so they notice how their tent sways gently between the trees, almost like being rocked gently to sleep and they did, rock gently to sleep in the tent. And after a week or so, of enjoying this exotic holiday seeing colourful birds, seeing different apes and other animals, taking plenty of photographs and writing down thoughts that came to mind. Then they took down their tents and travelled back home and they appreciated their own bed more than they had appreciated it in a long time. And they knew they had to do this more often as they relaxed down in their bed and drifted comfortably and deeply asleep.

TIME WAITS FOR NO MAN

Steps for increasing effectiveness of the story:

1. What do you want to achieve from reading this?

2. Think about one thing you have achieved today.

3. Say to yourself "When I read this story then…"

Alternative introduction:

"As I read this and begin to drift comfortably asleep, I don't know whether I will find myself drifting asleep more to the sound of my voice or the words I read, or perhaps to the spaces between the words. And as I drift comfortably asleep I'll just read this story to myself."

As you listen to me, you can begin to drift comfortably asleep and as you drift comfortably asleep I don't know whether you will fall asleep faster with the sound of my voice, with the words I use or perhaps the spaces between my words and as you fall asleep I'm just going to tell you a story.

This person finds herself walking through a strange land. She gazes out over that land as she is walking along and she can see floating land in the sky, she can see trees on that floating land, mountains on the floating land, she can see some of the floating land has waterfalls falling from that land down to the land below. She can notice that that floating land appears to be tethered to other floating lands. Almost like a matrix of floating lands in the sky with huge tethers between each bit of land and then there are points where there are tethers down to the ground. And the tethers don't appear to be manmade, they appear to somehow be just part of the environment. She had heard that in this land there were special magnetic rock, that there were areas where the magnetic rock would repel itself from the opposing magnetic force of the other rock and so these rocks were floating on a cushion of magmatism. She gazed out as far as the eye could see, she could see the gaps in the ground in the areas where the rocks had floated up into the sky. She didn't know what had caused the land to be this way. She could see lakes and the way the sun glistened on the surface of the lakes. She could see vast forests of tall trees with the occasional even taller tree poking out the top. Some areas where there was mist across the top of the forest, she could notice the colour of the sky, the clouds, birds flying high and she gazed out across this land and she had never been here before.

She was on a journey and had to find somebody. She didn't know what that person would be like, but she knew she would know when she found them. So, she walked down the hillside, walked down into the forest and started pushing through the forest. She could hear the sounds in the forest, the sounds of different animals, sounds of birds, sounds of her footsteps as she pushed on through the forest and while she pushed on through the forest she wondered who this person would be. She was just told to head west. She wasn't told how far or when she would meet that person, she just knew that she would recognise them and know that she had found them. She was told that they would happily talk to her and be very charming. She had something very important she needed to learn from them, so she continued to push her way through the forest. And as she pushed through the forest she wondered about how she could make sure she was staying heading west. She found this so much easier when she was out in the clearings where she could see the sky and be aware of her surroundings.

After sometime she managed to clear the forest and reach a lake. She created herself a raft and started paddling across the lake on that raft. She could hear the sound of the oar in the water as she pushed forward with her journey. She could hear the sound of the raft moving through the water and could smell the fresh water air and notice the subtle mist that hovered just above the water's surface. And so, she rowed across that lake. And at the far side of the lake she dragged her makeshift craft up onto the shore. Covered it over with some giant leaves in case she needed it and didn't want anyone to take it. She then carried on her journey west. And she came to a mountain and started to climb that mountain and as she climbed so trees thinned out until eventually she was above the trees and she continued climbing, continued climbing higher and higher. And she climbed up and over the mountain range and as she was on the other side of the mountain range, so she saw a dragon in the distance, circling round above some forest. And looking around she saw a bird of prey in another direction, flocks of birds flying in formations, sometimes birds launching themselves from the forest before landing elsewhere. She was aware of how much life was going on here, just going about its everyday business while she was on this quest to find this wise person.

She started down the mountain and found it much easier going down the mountain than going up. And as she was going down the mountain she noticed that there was running water down this side, flowing from the mountain and she started following that newly forming river which gradually turned into more of a torrent of water and waterfalls. And then at the foot of the mountain as the ground started levelling out so the water started slowing and the river started widening. And she felt it would be easier to follow the side of the river than to have to keep pushing forward through the forest. So, she followed this river. And after some time following this river, she saw an ornate bridge and either side of that bridge was a road and this road looked like it had been well kept and so it must be an important road leading somewhere. So, she went to that bridge and she saw that there was a man with a cane sitting on the bridge, just using the cane to prop himself up. And she greeted him and he greeted her back. Then he started talking to her and was charming with pleasant conversation. And she wondered if this was the wise man. She told him that she was on a mission. She had to find something of importance but she didn't know what, but she was told that the wise man would know and to just head west until she finds him. And he said "I have been sat here waiting to be found." She asked "What do you mean, 'you have been sat here waiting to be found,' are you lost?". He said "I am in exactly the right place for this moment.".

She asked him "How can you be wanting or needing to be found if you are not lost? Why don't you just go somewhere?". He said "I am somewhere, I am in the middle of somewhere and I would rather be here in the middle of somewhere than nowhere.". She asked him "But if you are somewhere and you are waiting to be found, how did you know to wait to be found, how did you know someone was looking for you?"

He replied "Somebody is always looking and nobody finds anyone, the only person who can find anyone is somebody, who is searching.".

And she found that his conversation was going through her head in some way. She didn't fully understand it at the moment, but it was so unusual that she assumed this must be the wise man.

He then said to her "Time stands still for no man.". And she thought that was an unusual thing for someone to say, of course time doesn't stand still.

He told her she is looking for time and when she has found time she will have found what she is searching for. She didn't understand and wanted to know how to find the time, she felt she didn't have time for this, she is looking for something and doesn't know what.

He explained that "You do know what, because I have told you, you just have to take the time and you need to discover it for yourself.". He said "All roads come to an end and you will have to decide which road you will want to follow to that end.".

And she replied "One road is probably the wrong road, the other road is probably right, how do I know which road to choose?".

And he said "You are right, one road is probably the wrong road and the road that is left is right.".

She thought to herself how this doesn't help at all, she is no clearer what road she should follow. He told her "You have all the answers. You just need to trust yourself and know that you know all the answers even if you don't know that you know them.".

And she thought to herself that this man is no help, she thought to herself that she is just going to wander down one of the roads and when she meets someone else she will ask them, maybe they can speak more sense, maybe this isn't the wise person really. So, she got up and left. And as she followed the left road she started to think about the interaction, started trying to process what he might have meant. And the road followed along the side of the river. And as she followed that road she allowed herself to get lost in thought, she found trains of thought stretching from one thing to another as she continued to walk, as she tried to process and make sense of what the man had said. And as she followed that road she could see across the river to the other road. And she could see that both roads looked like they were going the same way, just both on different sides.

And after many hours of walking it was starting to get dark. She had crossed mountains, she had walked miles, she felt she needed to sleep. So, she set up camp, lit a fire, had something to eat, took some time to meditate, to drift off in her mind, in her thoughts, to process her experiences, while she gazed at the flickering flames of the fire, aware of the flames dancing around, creating dancing light and shadows in the night and the sound of the water in the background, the sight of stars in the sky, the sound of rustling leaves as the wind blew a breeze. And she then settled down and drifted asleep and as she drifted comfortably asleep, so she started to dream. And while she dreamt, she replayed what that man had said, only in her dream the man didn't look like the man and he didn't quite say what he had said, but she knew this was a representation to learn from. And she imagined herself picking up a mirror, a handheld mirror and holding it out in front of her and looking at herself in that mirror and then suddenly being propelled faster and faster through space, getting faster and faster and faster. And noticing everything around her slowing down to the point where everything around her almost ground to a halt, where it was all going so slowly, that any movement was imperceptible and she looks to the left and she looks to the right and she looks up and she looks down and she looks around her and notices how everything has almost ground to a halt. And she looks forward again and notices that she can see her head turning in the mirror and everything in the mirror is happening in real time and yet, everything around her has slowed right down. And she knows that somehow this is all connected and yet, she doesn't know how.

She has this feeling like the sun is rising, a feeling of the warmth on her face, so she gradually opens her eyes while holding on to this dream and while she holds on to the dream she continues her journey. As she continues her journey she notices that the road on the other side of the river suddenly comes to an abrupt halt as it drops steeply into a gap left by one of the floating islands in the sky. And yet the road she is on just misses the edge of that gap and she notices how that river abruptly becomes a waterfall, pouring down into that gap. She looks up at that floating island, she looks down into the gap, she looks over at that other road and realises if she had been following that road it would have been a road to nowhere, that she would have to turn around and walk back again. And if she had just followed the river she would have to have tried to steer to the shore before the river turned into that waterfall and she continued walking along the road, looking down into the gap, looking up at the island, walking around that gap.

She passed the gap and carried on walking and she realised that wise man was actually wise in the first place, because what he had said was correct. He had said the path that was left was right. And she got up and left, following the left path. And she did it without any thought at all, she just decided to get up and decided to walk along that path, she didn't realise that she had done as he had said. It just happened instinctively, automatically. And after some time further of walking along this path she saw a palace, a palace that no-one lived in any longer and yet it looked like everyone had left just a day ago despite no-one living here for hundreds of years. And she walked into the palace grounds, walked through the palace grounds, past perfectly kept grounds of plants, flowers and shrubs. And as she entered the palace, so she could hear a ticking clock. And she walked instinctively towards the sound of that ticking clock, somehow, she felt that was what she was after, that she needed to find that ticking clock. And she came to a vast room in the middle of this palace with the ceiling so high she could barely see the top and in the middle was a circular table and on that table was an ornate beautiful clock. She went over to the clock, reached out and touched the clock and as she did, the ticking stopped.

And as the ticking stopped so she suddenly realised, time may not stand still for any man, but it has stood still for her. Then she touched the hands and slowly with her finger winds those hands back. And she doesn't know quite why she feels this is the thing to do as she winds those hands back and as she does she notices life coming back to the castle, to this palace, she notices people appearing, almost out of thin air. And then she reaches a point where as she is winding, she hears this slight click with the clock and she feels that this is the place where she is supposed to stop winding, so she stops winding moves her finger and hears the clock chime. And as the clock chimes, so all these people start milling around and moving as if life has returned to this palace. And someone is suddenly startled to see this woman they didn't see a moment earlier stood at the clock. And she knew with this that she had undone a curse that was brought upon her own land and that she had travelled from that was somehow connected through time and space with this palace and this clock. That in her own land, somehow time ground to a halt, everyone started disappearing as if they no longer existed and she got out of the land, but was aware that this problem was following her but not far behind, at the rate of one tick per tock and she couldn't really explain that, but she knew she was keeping ahead and had a sense that somehow there was a connection between these things. And she walked through all the people in the palace and went on her journey, able to enjoy this land more on her journey home. Knowing that she had changed her land and helped save the people in her land, just as much as she had helped to save the people in that palace. And when she eventually reached back to her land, she was gratefully received, she saw her loved ones, saw how happy she had made everyone. People had a vague sense that something had happened and now they were back and she looked forward to just going home, after a long journey, relaxing down and falling asleep.

Finding Happiness

Steps for increasing effectiveness of the story:

1. What do you want to achieve from reading this?

2. Think about one thing you have achieved today.

3. Say to yourself "When I read this story then…"

Alternative introduction:

"As I read this and begin to drift comfortably asleep, I don't know whether I will find myself drifting asleep more to the sound of my voice or the words I read, or perhaps to the spaces between the words. And as I drift comfortably asleep I'll just read this story to myself."

You can listen to this to relax and fall asleep, but it also contains additional therapeutic pattern to help those who want to lose weight.

Take a moment to close your eyes and begin to relax and you don't have to know how you are going to begin to relax, because you can relax in your own unique way. I don't know whether you will drift asleep deeper with the sound of my voice, the words I use, or the spaces between my words. And while you listen to me and relax I'll tell you this story.

And it is a story about a man who is sitting on a bench whilst one day, a monk walking past is just walking past in a relaxed way, being mindful of each step that he takes and as he walks past he notices this man sat on the bench. He notices that the man appears to be sad. And the man looks like he is perhaps depressed and not particularly motivated, so the monk decides to sit down on the bench and he turns to the man who is looking sad on the bench and he asks him "What is your story?".

And the man doesn't respond. And so, the monk calmly and firmly asks again "What is your story?".

And the way that the monk asked, helped jolt the man out of that world that he was in, in his mind. He shakes his head slightly as he brings himself round and he turns towards the monk, he sees the monk sat there and he starts to tell his story. He talks about how he had a beautiful wife, she was incredibly attractive, she seemed really sweet, but it turned out that she was bad for him. He did everything he could for her, he wanted her to be in his life, so he would do anything he could to try to make sure that that would happen, but what he found was that all she did was took from him. He felt good while he was with her, but then he ended up feeling bad when they were apart and he would end up craving wanting to be with her, even though he could see the harm she was doing to him. He spoke about how he didn't have much money, but he spent what he did have on his wife. That meant that then he didn't have enough money for the essentials that he needed. He spent money on fast cars, expensive items and he would end up feeling sad, or feeling like he might lose her, so he would want to spend lots of money on her. And whenever he felt sad, he would want to spend lots of money on himself to make himself happy. But then ended up feeling guilty and anxious and feeling sad again.

He ended up getting more and more in debt, with the debt growing larger and larger all the time. He described to the monk that it is like a sad, happy, guilt cycle. Where he would feel sad, spend lots of money to make himself feel happy and then he would feel guilty for all the money he spent, which would make him feel sad again. He spoke about how he finally left his wife. But now he feels that there is something missing in his life. Up to this point the monk had just been paying the man attention, just listening. Just absorbing what he is given. And then he leaned in and said to the man that it reminds him of the story of Hansel and Gretel, the story about the two of them finding the house made of sweets and they eat the sweets and they kind of know something is wrong with the house and they munch their way through the walls and they eat the sweets and the lady in the house keeps giving them more and more sweets and they just accept them and just keep eating and eating and eating, unaware that they are really being fattened up for the day when the witch can eat them. And the monk explained that the good thing about that story is that eventually they realised in time what was going on and they managed to turn things around so that they could escape and they could get out of there.

The monk explained that he could help the man to feel better. He could help the man to find a new path, to find a new way of filling that hole. He suggested that they go back to the man's house, to take a look at the house, so that he could share how he can help. And so, the man and the monk walked down the road back to the man's house. And when they arrived at the man's house the monk commented on the amount of junk that was in the house, all the stuff that the man had been buying over the years and the man commented that he finds it overwhelming. He looks at the task of having to clear the house, having to sell things, having to tidy up and all the different things he has to do and he just feels he has got too much on his plate. He is aware that he needs less on his plate. He needs to start somewhere small. He shared how he is uncomfortable with all of the clutter, that too much clutter gives him a bad feeling in his stomach and that he just can't relax.

So, the monk says that he will start to help with the clutter and that as the clutter clears, so the mind will clear also. And as the mind clears, so the man will begin to see things clearer and see where he can do and make different decisions and find a new path. And together they make a list of essential things which should be in the house, a list of the essential things he needs to do, a list of those things he needs to clear out and the things he needs to do to keep the house clear of junk in the future, so that he doesn't slip back into his old patterns, so that he takes on new patterns, new ways of being, so that he just follows these new patterns. And after the house is clear the monk and the man walk around the house, look at the clear kitchen, clear living room, clear dining room, gazing out of the window over the beautiful garden, clear and organised bedroom. All the rooms are organised and the monk tells the man he will teach him some helpful lessons for the future. He asks the man to go to the beach with him. The man complains, he said how he no longer has a car and so can't go to the beach with the monk. And the beach is only a few miles away, so the monk suggests that they walk and the man complained again. He complained that it is too much effort, it is too far to walk to the beach.

And anyhow he felt, the walk to the beach would be so boring. He is someone who would prefer to jump in the car and be somewhere as quickly as possible. And the monk firmly insists. He has got a way of kindly insisting things that encourages people to feel comfortable doing things that are for their own benefit. And the man and the monk walk to the beach and as they walk to the beach, the man notices the feeling of the breeze on his skin on his cheeks as they walk. He notices the sound of rustling leaves in the trees as he is walking down the path, notices the sounds of his footsteps and as he continues walking with the monk, he notices the feeling of his arms moving as they swing side to side. He notices the feeling of the ground beneath each footstep, he sees birds flying and perching in trees and landing and taking off of the path in front of him. He sees butterflies, insects and beetles. He sees so much he normally misses by speeding along in his car.

And every now and then the monk and the man strike up conversation, just general chat. And at some point, during the walk the man goes inside his mind and tells himself how he is beginning to enjoy the journey. He had always thought that the journey was the inconvenient part, that when you are going somewhere, the important part is where you are going. He had never considered that you can enjoy your journey to the destination. He always thought that you had to make the journey as quick as possible because it is just the journey and now he was beginning to realise that the journey doesn't have to be quick. The journey can be as long as the journey is. The important thing is enjoying that journey, as much as you would enjoy the destination. And sometimes plans change and you don't reach the destination you have aimed for and if you have enjoyed the journey, wherever you end up is okay. And the man gave a little smile and with this the monk looked over and said "It looks like you enjoy walking after all?".

And the man smiled some more and began to pick up the pace. Because the man really was enjoying the journey now, he really was enjoying walking. He never thought he would enjoy walking. But now, he is aware that he will probably walk far more often in the future. And as they arrive at the beach, so the path changes to stones and they walk on the stones and how each footstep sound changes, as they walk along the stones. And the man is aware of the sound of the sea, aware of looking out to the horizon, of other sounds around, of the sun in the sky, of the temperature. And they find somewhere to comfortably sit down on the beach. And the monk talked about how you choose your friends wisely. About how some people can be a problem and difficult to deal with and you don't want them to be on your plate, you don't want to have to deal with them. Whereas others make you feel good. Others make you happy and in doing so, they boost your health and your wellbeing. And they are the ones to spend time with. Those that make you healthy and feel good.

And the monk says to the man, while he is sat on the beach, "So take a moment to close your eyes and with your eyes closed, in a moment, I am going to reach over and I'm going to lift up your hand. And when I do, your hand is going to begin to get lighter and lighter and raise up more and more comfortably.".

And then the monk continued talking about something else and the man was feeling a bit uncomfortable with the uncertainty of not knowing when that hand will lift. He was trying to hear the monk. He could hear the sea, he could feel the breeze. As he sat there, waiting and waiting. And what he began to notice was, as that man sat their waiting, as time ticked by and the monk wasn't reaching over and lifting that arm. He began to shift inside himself. He began to shift from anticipation and uncertainty and uncomfortableness, waiting to know what is happening; to finding himself wander in his mind, wondering and finding himself becoming more comfortable and relaxed. And he noticed how he was relaxing deeper and deeper with each breath out and that as he was relaxing deeper and deeper with each breath out, so each breath out was stretching slightly longer than each breath in. And he began to notice that this is how to relax yourself. And while the man was beginning to relax and beginning to relax deeper and deeper, he mentioned that his brain constantly seemed to be on the go. It constantly seemed to be chattering and being drawn to things that upset him, drawn to things that he worries about the future, he worries about the past. He would tell himself that he was bored, he would say lots of negative things to himself.

And the monk explained, that is okay, it is just your brain thinking. So all you have to do is say to yourself that your brain is having a thought again and any time thoughts that you don't want are there just think to yourself "My brain is thinking again, my brain is thinking again, my brain is thinking again.".

Because, in reality that is the only truth in that moment, all it is, is a thought inside your mind. And so the man gave this some thought and he embedded this idea deep in his mind. This idea, deeply and unconsciously that his brain was thinking again and not to attach to it, not to give it any feeling, but to just acknowledge it for exactly what it is, that it is just the brain saying something. It isn't real-life, it is just the brain saying something, so there is no need for him to get emotional about that thinking, it is just the brain thinking, nothing more, nothing less, all he has to do is observe it, just as you can observe clouds floating by in the sky, you can observe sticks floating by on a stream, you don't have to try to grab every cloud, or to grab every stick, or give a judgement about every cloud or every stick. And you can just watch indifferently, just letting it pass by.

And while the man continued to sit quietly, the monk asked him to begin to observe your surroundings, begin to enjoy being in the moment, enjoy the inner journey and so the man began with his eyes closed, to pay attention to the water of the sea and the sounds the water makes. To pay attention to the sounds around him, the sound of the wind, to the feeling of the breeze, to the feeling of the ground beneath him. And he paid attention to his surroundings and he allowed himself to enjoy the moment. And almost like drifting comfortably asleep, he drifted into an inner journey, an inner journey of discovery, of personal growth and development. And he found himself in a forest. And everywhere he looked, everything looked the same and he thought to himself 'I now know where the saying 'I can't see the wood for the trees' comes from.' Because here in the forest he couldn't see anything, he couldn't make out anything, it all just looked the same. Most of the sounds echoed around the forest and he couldn't work out what direction they came from. And he walked through the forest, found his way through the forest, he figured out how to find his path and he had to cut his path through, to make it easier to walk. And he knew that by cutting his path through it would be easier to follow that path back. And after some time of cutting through, he found a shack deep in the forest. And in the shack, he found a chair and in that chair, he relaxed. And while he relaxed deeply in that chair, he drifted off into the most profound, deep, relaxing, sleep.

And in this deep relaxing sleep he began to have different thoughts spontaneously come up in his mind, like dreams coming up in his mind and he experienced many dreams in his sleep and while he experienced many dreams in his sleep, he found healthy alternatives to old habits. New and healthy ways of living life. And these new and healthy ways of living life embedded themselves in your neurology, as part of who you are.

And he gained insight about himself. He learned lessons, how to relax, how to control urges, how to look at the larger picture, rather than just deciding if something looks sweet it's going to be good. Instead, knowing that sometimes there is more to something than what you see on the surface. And then, as you comfortably drift deeper and deeper asleep, the man began to wake up. He found himself in that shack and walked back along the path he had come. And on his journey back he cut it a little wider, knowing that every time he visits this place and every time you listen to this, the path is easier and easier to follow because the path is cut wider and wider. And he knew he had found some answers to help him to become the person he wants to be.

And he found his way back and opened his eyes on the beach and noticed his arm was in the air. Just floating in the air and he slowly lowered his arm to his lap and then opened his eyes again and he felt that this was the first time he had truly opened his eyes, that the world he was living in before, the way he was living before, his eyes truly weren't open. And now his eyes were open. And he began to enjoy that feeling of knowing that changes have taken place in your mind and body. And he sat for a while talking to the monk, gaining lots of helpful information and all you need to know, before he went back home for the night, settled down and comfortably and relaxed, drifted off to sleep.

Finding Wisdom

Steps for increasing effectiveness of the story:

1. What do you want to achieve from reading this?

2. Think about one thing you have achieved today.

3. Say to yourself "When I read this story then…"

Alternative introduction:

"As I read this and begin to drift comfortably asleep, I don't know whether I will find myself drifting asleep more to the sound of my voice or the words I read, or perhaps to the spaces between the words. And as I drift comfortably asleep I'll just read this story to myself."

So, as you listen to me and you comfortably begin to fall asleep, I don't know whether you will find yourself drifting comfortably to sleep to the sounds of my words, to the spaces between my words, or just listening along to my voice in the background as you fall asleep. And while you fall asleep I am just going to tell you a story about a man who enjoyed going out to sea.

Every year he would go on a trip on a boat. His favourite thing was to swim with humpback whales. Every year he would go out on a boat, he would go out to sea on that boat and he would sit on that boat in diving gear and wait. And he would wait patiently and quietly, listening to the water lapping on the side of the boat, feeling the gentle rocking of the boat as he just gazes out over the water, feeling the sea breeze on his skin, noticing what the sky looks like, gazing out towards the horizon, scanning around the horizon, scanning the water for signs of the humpback whales arriving. And every year those humpback whales seem to arrive in this location.

And so, he just sits calmly and patiently and waits and not only does he like diving with the humpback whales, but he finds the entire experience calming and relaxing, just having patience, nothing to think about or worry about. Just waiting and relaxing. And then after some time, as the sun passes across the sky, he sees a little cloud appear from the ocean. And then the dark back of a humpback whale slides just above the surface of the water and back under again, so he drives the boat closer to the whales. And the closer he gets, the more he sees of what is there. He notices that there is an adult humpback whale and a juvenile humpback whale and he sees how calmly they are just swimming through the water. He drops the anchor and he drops into the water. He can feel that water flow into his wetsuit as he dives down under the water in his scuba gear. And he can see the size of those whales, see their slow graceful movements, hearing the whale calls. Just watching as those whales gracefully swim passed and watching how those whale's eyes appear to be so inquisitive, with such curiosity. And how the juvenile whale seems to want to come over to him and explore him. And the adult whale just keeps that juvenile at a bit of distance while assessing the diver and only after some assessing does the adult allow the juvenile and themselves to move closer.

They swim close enough for the diver to reach out with their hand and while their hand is outstretched, the juvenile swims in and rubs itself against his hand. And like all his past experiences, he feels this experience is an incredible experience, a moving experience, showing such intelligence in these whales, such love from the whales. He turns himself around weightlessly in the water, to keep tracking those whales as they swim comfortably around him. He enjoys this time in the water. Being in the water weightless with these whales, time seems to stand still. And after a while the whales take a deep breath and dive and he watches as they swim deeper and deeper and disappear out of sight. He then goes back to the boat, gets on the boat and steers the boat back to shore loving the experience he has just had.

And back on the shore, he goes back to the caravan that he is staying in, he always drives down here in a VW camper van so he goes back to the camper van he is staying in. He sits down and keeps a journal of his experiences. Not just a journal of the acts that he did and the behaviours, but a journal of his feelings, of how the experience made him feel and what that means to him.

And then, after writing his journal he sets up a camp just outside the caravan, just somewhere he can have something to eat on the seashore, a little campfire. And he enjoys the evening setting in, hearing the waves lashing on the shore, on the sand. Birds off in the distance, just sitting there enjoying the evening. Seeing the last of the suns' rays disappear and the stars in the sky. And as the evening draws on, he puts out the campfire, goes back into his camper van and settles down for the night to sleep. And as he drifts comfortably asleep, so he begins to dream and while he begins to dream, he begins to have a dream of himself sitting on a rose, sliding down a rose petal towards the centre of the rose and feeling the waxy touch of the petal under his hands as he slides and finding this feeling comfortable and safe and secure. The beautiful scent, the soft feeling of the waxy petal and he knows this dream has something to do with his daily experience. And he goes with the dream. And then he pops through the centre of the rose and finds himself sat at a desk in a chateau surrounded by woodland and mountains and finds that his hand is automatically writing as he gazes down at it and sees himself writing something unusual, he sees that he is writing some kind of a story.

He has this sense that he is writing a novel and he gets to a point where he gets drawn into that novel, into a scene where somebody is on a motorbike, going off-road, going around the outside of a mountain, following a mountain pass, following a dirt track. Riding that motorbike higher and higher up into the mountains. And he continues with the scene and there are a few areas where the motorbike skids and then catches the ground again and speeds off even faster and jumps at some areas and the bike is under full control of the motorcyclist. And that motorbike travels all the way to the top of the mountain. And the person on the motorbike is like a treasure hunter. And they are hunting for treasure that is somewhere here on the mountain and the person continues to write and as he continues to write he continues to be absorbed and drawn into this story, drawn into this story as this character discovers a temple high up here in this mountain.

And he picks a lock on the door to get into the temple, he walks into the temple and goes from the windy mountain's edge, to silence in the temple. He lights a torch and begins to explore in the temple and while he is exploring in the temple with the torch, so he can hear his footsteps echoing. He searches down one corridor and lights some torches as he goes and then searches down another corridor and then another. Noticing the way that his shadow and the light flickers on the walls, searching corridor after corridor. Until eventually, he comes to a dead end and at that dead end he sees what looks like a trap door on the ground. He prises open the trap door and climbs down a ladder going deeper and deeper under the temple and as he climbs deeper and deeper under the temple, so he realises he is climbing deeper and deeper down into the mountain, until eventually he comes out in a cave. And it appears to be a natural cave, it's not a man made cave. He thinks that maybe the temple was built over the cave on purpose. And he continues to explore this cave. And while he is exploring the cave, he starts to hear dripping water and gradually he starts to hear the distant sound of a waterfall and he continues exploring the cave. And while he is exploring the cave he is looking for some sign of a huge lost diamond, a legendary diamond.

And everything led him to this place and so he continues exploring and while exploring he finds a tunnel from the cave that looks man made and so he follows that tunnel and goes deeper and deeper until it comes out in a room and at the far side of that room is a huge locked door and he picks that lock and enters the room and in the middle of the room is a pedestal with a huge diamond sitting on it, lit up by natural light that seems to be channelled to the centre of the room through ice from the outside. And he goes over to the diamond and his plan is to take the diamond and then sell it, but as he reaches the diamond he sees a book. He picks up the book and starts reading and as he starts reading so he learns that this diamond is placed here to bring peace to the land and that there is darkness that will be unleashed if this diamond gets removed. And anyone who discovers this diamond has to look inside themselves and decide what is more important, peace across the land, keeping the darkness at bay, or having the diamond and making lots of money? And he thinks about it. He doesn't know what this darkness is, he can't imagine a real darkness, that would be the thing of legends and myths, so it must be a legend or a myth, it can't be real. The book ends by saying that he is to put his hands on either side of the pedestal where there are two symbols and to close his eyes and that will teach him that everything in this book is true. He thinks to himself that it all sounds ridiculous, but it takes no effort to put your hands on the side of something and to close your eyes for a moment, to prove that it is ridiculous.

So, he puts his hands on either side of the pedestal and he closes his eyes and initially he doesn't feel anything and then he starts feeling a tingling at his hands, that starts in his fingers, or perhaps his palm and eventually starts moving up to his wrists, his arms, his shoulders and in to his body and a warmth, a comfort and he has a sense of a light, a purple light, as if it is given off by the diamond in front of him. He can see it with his eyes closed, he can sense that purple light shining on his face, passing into his head, his body, absorbing into him, this purple light, passing in to him, filling him up with this purple light. And he starts to have a feeling of serenity, of peace, of love, of wonder and curiosity, a sense of a connection with the world around him, a sense of what is important. And he finds it a powerful, emotive experience. And then he removes his hands from the pedestal and in a moment the experience passes and he opens his eyes and he is just there with that pedestal with that diamond and he realises that the diamond needs to stay where it is and needs to be protected. And he leaves and seals the entrance to that room and he leaves and seals every entrance behind him and leaves that mountaintop temple and seals the door and then motorbike's back down the mountain with that serene feeling, that learning, that knowledge he gained that will stay with him forever.

And the writer had this feeling that the story was coming closer to an end, as the man found himself with the petals falling down around him, gently floating down to the ground, as he was sat in the middle of these giant rose petals, just falling around him, comfortably, calmly, as he drifted from this dream into a deeper more comfortable, healing, relaxing, sleep.

GIRL ON A COUNTRY WALK

Steps for increasing effectiveness of the story:

1. What do you want to achieve from reading this?

2. Think about one thing you have achieved today.

3. Say to yourself "When I read this story then…"

Alternative introduction:

"As I read this and begin to drift comfortably asleep, I don't know whether I will find myself drifting asleep more to the sound of my voice or the words I read, or perhaps to the spaces between the words. And as I drift comfortably asleep I'll just read this story to myself."

As you rest there and begin to comfortably fall asleep, you can hear my voice in the background and as you hear my voice in the background so you can begin to drift off asleep and I don't know whether you will fall asleep faster with the sound of my voice, or with the words that I use, or whether it will be with the spaces between my words.

As you fall asleep I'm just going to tell you a story about a girl in a meadow and this girl grew up in the countryside and she loved it in the countryside and every day she wandered out into the countryside and she looked forward to going outside whatever the weather and she looked forward to going outside and being part of nature and enjoyed going outside and making the most of her day.

And on this day, she has gone outside and wandered along from her property and she wanders along and finds her way to a chalk bridleway and there are patches of green grass down the centre of the bridleway and this bridleway has been used for hundreds and hundreds of years and so it is worn down and the chalk is clearly visible down both sides, with chalk and flint and some other stones and mud. It is a nice dry and sunny day. And she walks down this bridleway gazing out at the fields on either side, looking up and noticing the blue sky, noticing wispy clouds in the sky, she pays attention to notice how fast the clouds are moving and in what direction and she tries to work out whether it looks like the clouds are moving in the same direction as the breeze that she can feel, or whether the clouds are moving in a different direction and perhaps the wind up there is heading in a different direction to the wind down here. And little things that she found curious. And she looked out to the left and right over the different fields and she could see that in the fields were different crops and in one field was the most beautiful yellow and smelled gorgeous and another field was green and another field was purple and full of lavender. And she could see the different butterflies, different bees, different creatures enjoying the different environments, the different fields.

And she was walking past these fields to go to some hills in the distance. The hills didn't have use like the fields did. Sheep grazed on the fields and kept the grass short and she wanted to go and sit on the grass on the hill looking over the countryside and so she walked all the way to those hills. And as she walked towards the hills, so she found a little village area she walked through and while she walked through the village with cobbled roads, the most beautiful houses, the most colourful flowers, she felt herself drawn in to the smell of a rosebush. And she stopped and lingered near that rosebush, taking in the smell of the roses, enjoying that smell, watching the bees landing on the roses, getting on with their day, noticing the way the roses in the bush moved and swayed in the breeze, just enjoying that. And the interesting thing about these roses was the way they didn't have thorns and so she picked one of the roses to take with her.

And as she carried on walking she would put the rose under her nose to enjoy the smell from time to time and she would gaze up with delight and a smile on her face with a feeling of happiness while she walked through this beautiful village heading towards those hills. And she saw different flowers, she would stop and smell them. And as she would mindlessly walk through the village while gazing around, she would find herself touching petals of different flowers, noticing the smooth and silky, slightly waxy feeling of the petals, enjoying that feeling of the petals while walking along. She was aware of the warmth of the sun on her skin and on her face, the way it was warming her cheeks and the breeze in her hair.

And as she passed out the other side of the village continuing her journey, she noticed a cat that joined her, a little black and white cat. She could hear it meowing as she neared. And she didn't approach it, it approached her; which is the way it should be. It jumped down off a wall and ran over to her legs and weaved itself around her legs, around one leg and over a foot and between her legs and back around the other leg, weaving itself in a figure of eight around and between her legs, rubbing its body on her legs. And she carried on walking and the cat started walking beside her, following along wanting to walk with her and she was nearing the meadow, nearing the hill and it wanted to walk along with her and so she just let it walk along with her for a while, she knew that it knew its territory, it knew where it was and knew where it wanted to go, she wasn't taking it anywhere, it was deciding what it wanted to do and she knew where it had found her and so she knew it could follow her back to there afterwards. And as she reached the meadow and climbed up the hill she settled down on the grass and could feel the cool grass beneath her and enjoyed the feeling with her fingertips and the palm of her hands of the grass beside her. She relaxed back and the cat climbed onto her lap, curled up and rested and started purring and so she gently started stroking that cat with one hand while with the other hand she started reading a book, holding and reading a book. She liked to let her mind drift off. She liked to be lost in a book and so she sat there on that hillside, taking some time to feel nature, feel being part of nature while reading a book and stroking that cat.

And then after a while of reading, she laid down on her side with the cat laying down beside her, she just stroked the cat gently, with the cat purring, just listening to the surroundings, listening to the birds in the distance, listening to sheep bleating, listening to other sounds while resting there. The sound of the breeze, the sound of rustling leaves of trees. Enjoying the warmth of the sun. The comfort of the warmth of the sun, the breeze in her hair and she just rested there. And she found her mind drifting and wandering so comfortably and calmly and felt so peaceful.

After some time, she decided it was time to go on a wander, so she wandered back towards the village, to guide that cat back to the village and after guiding that cat back to the village she decided to take a different route, she turned down a different path, wandering down to the river. And as she wandered down to the river she could gradually hear that river getting louder and louder as she got closer and closer. She knew it was quite a rough river, there was a lot of spray from the river and she liked being down by the river, especially on warm sunny days with the feeling of the spray and so she walked down by the river and she could see how rough it was and although it was rough, it was shallow and safe, it was just the layout that made it appear quite rough and sound rougher than it probably really was.

And she sat on a rock beside the water and took her shoes off and put her feet into the water to just enjoy that feeling of the water rushing through her feet and the sound of that water and smelling that fresh water and noticing how that water is so cool compared to the warm sun. And the kind of tickling feeling of the running water. And she sat there for a while on that rock, enjoying that flowing, running, rough water. Then after a while, she walked through the water to get to the other side of the river and could feel that rough water rising up above her ankles, tickling just above her ankles as it bubbled around her feet. And she got to the other side and walked barefoot into the grass, feeling the way the grass felt compared to the water and the rocky bed under the water. And she decided to sit down on the grass, let her feet dry in the sun. And just enjoy this day out.

And she sat there, drifting off in a daydream, having her own little reverie, allowing herself to become lost in thought. Thinking pleasant thoughts and dreams and aware of how much she just enjoys the simple life, that these things are the most precious things in life, being out in nature, being one with the world around you, connected with nature. She thought to herself that it isn't all about possessions, a good book is all you need, a good book and the natural outdoors. And after a while she decided it would be good to start heading home. Make sure she will be home in time for tea, in time for something to eat before bed, so she walked to a path, put on her shoes and took a different route back walking along this path that had the same chalky effect from all of these chalk hills around the area, walking in to some woodland, enjoying her time through that woodland, noticing deer in the woods, hearing birds, noticing woodpeckers, glancing a butterfly. Working her way through the woods and after coming out of the woods she goes over a bridge that takes her to the other side of the river, follows the path which takes her round in front of that village and continues along the path and follows the path all the way back towards her home. She walks past those fields and decides to slow down and pick some of the lavender and carries on walking and enjoys the smell of the lavender, enjoys the smells from the other fields, gazes off and notices a bird circling overhead so gracefully and wanders all the way back home.

On arriving home, she takes her shoes off, settles down and has something to eat. Then after a while she decides it is time to go to bed, so she goes to bed, lies down and as she drifts comfortably asleep, she allows her mind to wander to her journey that day and in her mind's eye she follows that journey, she follows that journey along the side of the fields, she follows the journey around to the village, she thinks about that rose, what it smelled like, what it felt like, she follows the journey around to finding that cat and making friends with that cat. And as she is falling asleep she feels a little smile coming to her face. She finds that as she falls asleep, she doesn't try to fall asleep, she just thinks about things make her feel good, things that make her feel lost in thought, things she would like to think about as she drifts off to sleep and she thinks about those things and she naturally and comfortably falls asleep.

And she has a sense of that little cat, what it was like to stroke the cat, to chill out with that cat while reading the book, to be listening to sheep and other animals, to be enjoying some time up on that hillside. She recalls what it was like to be dangling her feet in the water and listening to that rough water bubbling away. And she recalls her walk back, the deer she saw in the woods.

And as she drifts comfortably asleep, she rolls over slightly and notices the smell of lavender still on her fingers and recalls picking the lavender on the way home just before she saw that bird high in the sky. She starts to wonder what kind of experiences she is going to have tomorrow and what she will fall asleep dreaming about tomorrow. And she drifts comfortably and falls asleep.

Legend of the Book of Knowledge

Steps for increasing effectiveness of the story:

1. What do you want to achieve from reading this?

2. Think about one thing you have achieved today.

3. Say to yourself "When I read this story then…"

Alternative introduction:

"As I read this and begin to drift comfortably asleep, I don't know whether I will find myself drifting asleep more to the sound of my voice or the words I read, or perhaps to the spaces between the words. And as I drift comfortably asleep I'll just read this story to myself."

As you listen to me and begin to comfortably fall asleep I don't know whether you will drift off asleep faster to the sounds of my words or to the sound of my voice, or whether you will drift off to sleep faster to the spaces between my words. And as you comfortably begin to fall asleep you can allow your eyes to close as you listen to me talking in the background

And while I talk in the background as you fall asleep I'm going to tell a story about a person out on a horse one day. And this person enjoyed going out horse riding, they lived near some vast open countryside with sprawling meadows, a few rolling hills and some woodland and they enjoyed going out regularly exploring this countryside.

And one day they were out exploring the countryside, sitting on the back of the horse as it rode out of their farmland and started riding off into that countryside. They could feel the horse between their legs, the warmth of the horses' neck at their hands. The feeling of the movement as the horse walked. The sound of the horses' hooves on the floor and they could feel the air on their skin and notice what the sky looked like while the afternoon sun travelled across the sky. Noticing the way the breeze affected the grass and wild plants. Seeing birds flying in the sky and just enjoying a comfortable ride out into the countryside. And after a few hours of riding they stopped for a while, gave the horse something to drink and the horse started eating some grass and they could hear that sound of the horse taking mouthfuls of grass, while they stopped and had something to eat and drink as well. They thought about how calm and how pleasant these riding experiences are. Just an opportunity to get away from everything for a while. And while they sat there letting their horse rest and eat, they rested and let their mind wander. Just drifting to pleasant thoughts and ideas and after a while they continued their journey on that horse. They were heading to a lake which is down near the woodland.

And they continued on that horse all the way down towards the lake. And as they approached the lake, they noticed how the air temperature changed slightly, the breeze was a little cooler as the air blew across the surface of the water before reaching their face. They noticed how the sun was beginning to set and they decided, now would be a good time to put up a tent. Start a fire, cook some food and settle down for the night. So, they put up a tent by the edge of the lake, they created a small fire just in front of the tent. They tied the horse to a nearby tree giving plenty of rope for the horse to roam around, to lie down, to walk over to the lake, to have a drink and they also gave some extra food to the horse. They felt that the horse was almost like family. They made themselves some food on the fire, had themselves a drink and just sat in the entrance to the tent, just being, not doing anything particular, but just being. They sat in that entrance of the tent, hearing the crackling fire as it started dying down to embers, feeling the warmth given off by the fire as it died down to embers. Seeing the way the moonlight was dancing on the surface of the lake and the stars they could see in the sky. And as they gazed up at those stars, noticing the way they were twinkling, noticing the occasional shooting star, they almost heard whiz past, they just found the experience so calming, so relaxing.

This opportunity to have some peace, some quiet, some time to separate from the hustle and bustle of daily life, of jobs they have got to do, of different tasks, of different responsibilities, just being able to focus on being in the here and now, being in this moment, just enjoying being here. And they could hear the lake very gently lapping on the shore. And they continued to feel that breeze, mixed with the warmth of the fire and hear the sound of their horse lying down, not far away. And then after a while, they began to feel tired, they began to want to drift comfortably asleep, so they lay back in their tent, they did the tent up and began to drift comfortably asleep. And while they were drifting comfortably asleep they could hear the breeze on the outside of the tent, hear the sounds of nature outside the tent, while relaxing and drifting and falling asleep for the night. Then in the morning, they were awoken by the sounds of birds, by the glow of sunlight making the tent seem to glow on the inside with light coming from all directions. And as they started reorienting to the sounds, to the sights, they began to notice movement of the side of the tent with the breeze. They opened the entrance to the tent, breathed in that fresh morning air, there was still just the slightest warmth from the fire, from the embers that had burnt down. Their horse was already up eating some grass, appearing very chilled.

And they came here because they had heard that there was a book on the island in the centre of this lake. And they wanted to go and try to find it, because they had heard that this book taught secret knowledge and wisdom, which got them curious. They had heard legends about this area before, but they had never thought that the actual location was somewhere so close they could check it out for themselves to see if it was real, or at least, check it out and discover that it is just a legend. They got themselves a raft that inflated, which they had carried on the horses' back. They placed it down on the edge of the lake, they inflated the raft and left their tent all set up. They saw no need to take the tent down and they got into the raft, pushed away from the shore and started rowing across the lake towards the island in the centre. There were a few trees on the island, some bushes on the island. Occasionally birds nest on the island and birds would often congregate on the island because it was away from the edge of the lake where any foxes or other predators could get them. And they rowed out into the lake. They could hear the sound of the oar as they pushed the water behind them and feel the weight of the water as they push the oar back through the water and the way the raft gets pushed forwards with each push of the oar. They noticed how the air smelled so fresh just above the water as they continued rowing in the morning sun. After about twenty minutes of rowing they arrived at the island, rowed the boat a little bit up onto the island and climbed off.

They then pulled that raft out of the water and up onto the bank of the island. They didn't want to lose the raft and have to swim back to the other side. They started to explore this small island, looking for any clue as to whether there was actually a book hidden somewhere here. They explored around the outside of the island first and then started walking slightly inward and explored in a circle again and then walked slightly inward again and explored in a circle again. Then they noticed a carving in a tree of an arrow.

They followed the direction that the arrow was pointing, they didn't know how far they should follow it, what clue they would see, or whether the arrow was even related to what they were searching for or whether they would even find anything and if the arrow didn't lead to anything they could just go back and continue circling as they had been. And as they walked, looking around, gazing around with their senses open, looking for anything that could be a clue, they tripped over something on the ground and then found that it was a small little stone that had been carved but had now grown over with grasses and mosses and vines and so pretty much blended in with the surroundings. And that was pointing in a different direction.

They started walking in that direction, they thought, two clues mean they must be on to something even if they don't know what and that they definitely must be clues because the first pointed in one direction and the second was on the route of the first clue. As they walked, they arrived at a tree which seemed to be directly in their way. They thought about walking around it and carrying on walking until they find a clue, but they wondered, what if the tree is the clue? Why would you bury something, or have something somewhere, where you have a marker pointing straight at a tree to it, wouldn't you have the marker positioned to point slightly past the tree? They took some time to analyse the tree to see what they could learn. The size of the tree matched up with whatever it was that was buried a few hundred years ago, it looked like the tree was a few hundred years old like it may have been planted at the same time.

They looked around the base of the tree, trying to find any clue, then they broadened out slightly from the base of the tree and circled around trying to find any clue. Then they got down on their hands and knees and started stroking the ground with their hands trying to see if there were any clues. With their hand they noticed a slight lump on the ground. There were no other lumps, the rest of the ground seemed normal, just grass and mud, but this lump seemed more solid. It could have just been a bit of the trees' roots, but they decided to uncover it to take a better look. As they uncovered it they discovered that it was a small metal handle, a handle to a trapdoor which they discovered was buried just slightly under the mud with just the handle poking out. They tried to pull the trapdoor open, but it didn't pull open easily because of all the roots of the grass and other plants growing over the top of it. Using a penknife, they carefully cut at the roots around the trapdoor, lifted the trapdoor open and saw some narrow steps leading down diagonally underneath the tree.

They thought to themselves that this definitely seems like a clue. They squeezed down the narrow stairs, going deeper and deeper under the tree. They used a torch to see and they noticed that it opened up into a cavern that appeared to be supported by some kind of stone structure and the tree was growing above and around the arched stone structure. And in the centre was a pedestal with an old ornate book sitting on top of it. They walked over to the book, they thought about whether they should take this book with them or leave this book here. They decided if it has been here this long, perhaps it is best to keep it here rather than take it, but they did think that maybe someone else in the future would come here and take it. So, they opened the book and started reading. And what they read was that this book was placed on the site of a spring. A spring that filled the lake. And the whole island was built on top of that spring and the water seeps up through the island and starts to fill the lake around the edges of the island. They continued reading and learned that this spring is a fountain of youth. The water in the lake leads to youthfulness, to healing, to wellbeing. And the newer and fresher the water is, the more effective the healing properties are. So, the healing is greatest at the spring.

They read that this led to problems, people started fighting over the spring, they were fighting over wanting this water, over wanting power and wanting to live forever and be fit and healthy forever. And as the water, over time, loses its effectiveness it was decided to build an island over the top of the spring so that by the time the water has filtered through and spread out into the lake quite a bit of time has passed and anyone drinking the water at the edge of the lake will get some healing benefit, but they are unlikely to live forever because the potency is significantly reduced. They had to stop it being possible for people to drink from the spring. And as time went on people were initially kept away from the area. There were legends and rumours about this spring, this fountain of youth, but as future generations couldn't see that there was any evidence of this, they just assumed it was a legend. And the book was left here to tell the story by the last survivors from the fountain of youth who had been drinking the water and who made the decision to stop drinking the water after they saw that it had drifted in to legend.

The person felt that perhaps someone else might come and do the wrong thing by this message but having this book in any other location would lead people to investigate and try and find this spring, would ruin the environment, would dig up the lake, until eventually they would find the spring and someone would likely try and make money selling that spring water. So, they closed that book, kept it where they found it, they covered over the trap door after they left it.

They know it wouldn't take long for nature to reclaim the top and clean everything up. They added a bit more dirt this time to hide the handle. They removed the waypoint stone marker so that it wasn't pointing to the tree anymore and they left the arrow on the tree and they went back and rowed back over the lake. The sun was beginning to set and so before they journeyed home, they decided to camp for one more night. They checked on their horse, had a little talk with their horse, gave their horse some food and rode them around a little bit before settling down for the night in the tent, drifting comfortably and relaxed asleep, before heading home in the morning.

LIFE AS AN OAK TREE

Steps for increasing effectiveness of the story:

1. What do you want to achieve from reading this?

2. Think about one thing you have achieved today.

3. Say to yourself "When I read this story then…"

Alternative introduction:

"As I read this and begin to drift comfortably asleep, I don't know whether I will find myself drifting asleep more to the sound of my voice or the words I read, or perhaps to the spaces between the words. And as I drift comfortably asleep I'll just read this story to myself."

Life as an Oak Tree

As you listen to me, you can begin to relax and as you begin to relax so you can start the process of falling asleep comfortably. And while you begin to drift off asleep comfortably I'll continue talking to you in the background and as I talk to you in the background, you don't have to pay any attention, you can just let yourself drift off asleep.

And as you listen to me, beginning to relax deeply, you can imagine what it is like to be born as a tree. You can start life a thousand years ago. And you start off like a tiny twig sticking out of the ground with just a couple of leaves on top of your head. And it is interesting, life on these time scales. What it is that you have seen, what you have witnessed and experienced, changes, events over time. And as you begin to grow, you sway in the wind, you experience the seasons, you experience spring, heading in to summer, with the explosion of colour and growth and warmth and light. As this moves in to autumn and the colours turn rusty and the temperature cools and perhaps there is a little bit more wind. And the days are shorter and the sun never rises quite so high above the horizon. And the growth of other plants and grass, slows down, as the seasons move on to winter. And you feel packed comfortably in ice and snow, with just a white glow around you. And the crunching sound of people and animals walking in the snow. Trees being bare of their leaves, waiting for the spring. Then as the snow melts and spring arrives and you notice those frosty mornings in early spring where cobwebs take on a beautiful shimmer, look across fields of grass as light glistens on water droplets caught in the webs. And the weather warms up quickly, creating a mist above the fields. And a beautiful sunrise in the distance.

And you experience these seasons year after year, just like clockwork. Where spring leads to summer, leads to autumn, leads to winter, leads back to spring. You see the increase in animals and the decrease in animals. The increase in other plant life and the decrease in other plant life. The sun rising higher in the sky and then rising lower in the sky. Days getting longer and then days getting shorter. While you continue to grow taller and you start off growing flexibly in the wind and gradually as you grow taller you become sturdier. And while you become sturdier, you become better able at weathering harsh weather. And it is nice to remain flexible as well. And you see that young couple sitting beneath your leaves when you are just a young tree. They carve their names into the bark and a love heart, they gaze out over the meadow, over to a small town with a church in the distance. And you can be aware of that church bell ringing and that couple enjoying sitting in the shade of your leaves as they rustle and move in the breeze.

And throughout the years, that couple comes back to sit beneath your leaves and they climb up into your branches and they sit on your branches and they chat and just enjoy each other's company. And year after year they return. You notice them getting older gradually. Year after year they return. And after a few years, different couples start coming along, sitting in the shade of your leaves. Starting their own relationships, enjoying their time with you here. Gazing out over that old English town over there. Listening to the church bells in the distance. As you continue to grow taller and wider and get a fuller head of leaves, you weather harsh storms that roll in from time to time. And incredibly warm weather and heavy rains and very dry weather and you experience all sorts of weather. And yet, you just stand strong, stand firm, just watching as time goes by. And as the years turn into decades and decades begin to turn in to centuries, you notice how people change, you notice how their clothing changes, you notice that the houses people are living in change. The number of people changes. You notice so much history.

And as the centuries move on, so you relax deeper and deeper into where you are, stretching out those roots, deeper and deeper, wider and wider. Growing those leaves more fully, being aware of different buildings being erected, of changes from medieval times to industrial times, to Victorian dress, noticing when the people went through a renaissance time and artists would come and sit in the shade of your leaves and would paint the most beautiful pictures of the scene before them. And you would find your mind wandering, drifting and wandering, because you are only able to be stuck in this one place.

You get to see time passing by, you get to see painters and more recently, photographers, you get to see how towns and cities change, you get to see how the weather changes, month after month, year after year. You get to see lovers sitting under your leaves, you get to have people stealing a kiss. You get to share in secrets and wonder and intrigue, but you always wonder what it would be like to move, what it would be like to be somewhere else. To be able to move and have a different perspective. To be able to fulfil your curiosity. And you find your mind wandering and imagining what it would be like to drift and float through space and time. Drifting and floating through space and time, comfortably into another location, seeing from another location. And you wonder what that will be like.

And you enjoy some time imagining what it would be like to be in a different location, what insights you gain, what you learn there. You wonder what it would be like to have the ability to move from your spot. What it would be like to be one of these people who you have seen. And you enjoy being a tree, growing taller and wiser with each passing year. And then when the time is right, you find yourself as a tree, almost drifting in to a hibernation, as one winter approaches, just conserving your energy as you drift comfortably inside, like you have done hundreds of times before over the years, drifting inside, creating an inner world of dreams, drifting in a dream where you can drift inside and enjoy dreaming and drifting and sleeping for a while, knowing you will awaken again in the spring.

Life on Mars

Steps for increasing effectiveness of the story:

1. What do you want to achieve from reading this?

2. Think about one thing you have achieved today.

3. Say to yourself "When I read this story then…"

Alternative introduction:

"As I read this and begin to drift comfortably asleep, I don't know whether I will find myself drifting asleep more to the sound of my voice or the words I read, or perhaps to the spaces between the words. And as I drift comfortably asleep I'll just read this story to myself."

So, as you listen to me and begin to comfortably fall asleep, I don't know whether you will fall asleep faster with the sounds of my words, with the spaces between my words, or whether it will be with the words that I use. And as you fall asleep, so I will talk in the background and tell a story.

And I'll tell a story about a man who was one of the first to start colonising Mars. And there are only a handful of people who have started to colonise Mars. They have been creating a domed Martian base that is made with see-through aluminium that looks just like glass.

One morning this man was out on his run, as he does every morning, where he runs around the inside of the dome. He does a number of laps around the inside of the dome and while he is running, he finds he still hasn't got used to the fact that it feels different to when running on Earth, that each stride launches you further and is more effortless than on Earth. And so, because of this reduced gravity here, he has to run and exercise for a couple of hours each day to make sure that he keeps himself fit and healthy and keeps his bones fit and healthy. And while he runs around the inside of the dome he often finds himself gazing out of the dome, gazing through the triangular windows, gazing through that see-through aluminium that looks like glass. And while he does, he sees the red planet, he sees how it looks kind of familiar, but alien at the same time, but there is no life out there on the surface. It looks like places he had been to train on Earth before his trip here. And occasionally vast dust storms appear and everything gets plunged into darkness inside the dome and they have to use artificial light.

The dome is powered by many different power sources, they gather some of the wind and when dust settles, that tips the propellers and also then powers them, because the propellers are designed almost like they have little cups on them, they are designed to be really smooth and non-stick and channel any dust that lands on a propeller blade down to the cup at the end, so any dust landing on a blade slides down the blade towards the cup adding weight to the end of the blade tipping that blade and making that blade move down which empties the cup and as the cup on the next blade then fills up, that does the same, it tips the blade down, moving that blade and emptying the cup and so it continues. So, the blades capture wind to create electricity, but even in dust storms they can generate electricity. They use solar panels and have a huge array of solar panels, but the panels need wiping down after dust storms and during dust storms they are almost totally ineffective.

And they have been creating other fuel with the resources found on Mars. Part of their job is to do the research to make sure it will definitely be self-sustaining for more colonists to come here. And the man continues running around the inside of the dome, noticing how the sun has a very slightly purple hue as it is near the horizon. And inside the dome is a comfortable temperature and yet he is aware that outside the dome, even though it doesn't look cold it is actually way below zero. And after his running around the dome, he then does some more exercises before having some breakfast. And after breakfast it is his job to get on with some work and he gets into his spacesuit and walks into an airlock as the door shuts behind him, the section is then changed in pressure, he then opens the airlock and walks out onto the Martian surface and inside the spacesuit is a speaker connected to a microphone which is on the outside of the spacesuit so that he can clearly hear what it would sound like to be walking on Mars without the spacesuit on. He can hear his footsteps, he can hear when the breeze blows against the microphone. They have been experimenting with attempts to create life that can survive on Mars, with the plan that in centuries time, they can perhaps terraform Mars, but if they can create life and plants that they can eat, that can grow in Martian soil and the Martian atmosphere, they don't have to do all that inside the dome, they can maximise space by doing all of that outside of the domes.

And so, he goes over and chisels away at some bits of stone and takes samples and puts them in a bag. He chisels away at other stone, takes samples and puts them in a bag. He then goes to different locations where experiments are being carried out, where seeds have been planted. And the seeds are unable to be watered because the water just evaporates or freezes depending on what they do to the water. Or the water has to be far too salty for it to be liquid. So, they have to figure out what areas a hardy plant could grow. So, he goes over and looks at one area, nothing is growing there, so he marks that down. He goes to another area and it is the same, nothing is growing there. He goes and checks out another area and nothing is growing there. And then he checks in an area that is just inside a nearby cave, just in the mouth of a cave. He notices the tiniest of little bits of life. He notices some small leaves just poking out of the ground and somehow this is able to survive here. Perhaps because it is just out of the radiation, maybe in this cave area there is a little bit more moisture just under the ground, near enough for the roots to reach. Whatever the reason, there seems to be a bit of life here.

So, they take a sample of this bit of soil that they can analyse and try and work out what is different about this specific location. And if it works out in this location, the difficulty is that it is not so scalable because they can't just grow all the plants in caves and the plants will probably still need some kind of sunlight for photosynthesis. But, something he notices while he is checking in the cave, is that there is something on the walls. It looks like it is a bit slimy and it is something that is perhaps growing without photosynthesis. He doesn't know whether it is something that is naturally

Martian, or something that has got there from Earth. But he knows it is not part of the experiment and he knows if he hadn't walked into the cave just that little bit further than usual and hadn't been nearer to the side than usual he wouldn't have noticed that there was this stuff on the walls. He knew that on Earth there are some things that survive without photosynthesis and so he takes a sample that he can take back to be analysed back in the lab, back in the dome. He carries on his rounds to the other locations and doesn't find anything else and so starts to make his way back to the dome.

He quite likes being out on the Martian surface. He doesn't mind being in the dome, looking out over the Martian's surface, but he feels trapped because he feels that the dome is like a barrier. He knows he is on a different planet, he doesn't feel trapped when he is walking on the Martian surface. He enjoys going on expeditions, he enjoys exploring valleys, vast ravines, tall mountains and ancient volcanos. He enjoys having that sense of awe and wonder that everything is so big at times. That you don't feel like you are trapped somewhere. He enjoys at night, seeing the most beautiful view of the night sky, views you could never get on Earth. And so, he heads back to the dome, he shares his findings and then he starts working on that discovery, on that life he found and in a lab he takes a small amount and extracts some of the DNA. He finds that it is subtly different in how it is made up compared to DNA he is used to seeing under an electron microscope. And so they analyse the DNA in more detail and it doesn't quite match how DNA is done on Earth and he realises that there is a very good chance that this isn't Earth life and that they had thought there was no life on Mars and that there certainly wasn't any life on the surface of Mars and yet, near the surface where it is sheltered from solar rays, from radiation, inside caves, there is this life. Slimy kind of life that just seems to grow on the rocks. And they analyse this life and see that it seems to produce a chemical that can erode the rocks ever so slightly and that erosion feeds the life. The erosion creates chemicals that the life can feed on. And then the carbon dioxide in the atmosphere feeds the life further and the life doesn't need photosynthesis, it can just live on, eroding the rocks. This type of life, likely makes its own caves over millions of years by just gradually eroding the rock and multiplying and continuing to erode the rock. He finds this a fascinating discovery, that somehow this life can live off of the rocks, just by creating a simple chemical reaction on the surface that dissolves the rocks, that gets some iron out of the rocks, some oxygen out of the rocks, uses the carbon from the atmosphere and it seems to be a very slow growing organism.

They continue to study this life and now realise that whatever they do, they can't mess with the ecosystem too much because there is actually life here on Mars where they thought there was none and if they mess with it too much then they may interfere with the life that is here without realising what they have interfered with. This man found that today was probably the most exciting day he had had here on the red planet. Every day had been the same, get up, exercise, eat, get in your spacesuit, go out exploring, go and do your rounds, do a bit more exploring, spend a few hours typing up reports about your findings, have a bit of social time and then go to bed. Although he was fine doing this every day, this was something new and exciting, this was a dream that humanity had had for years, of finding life on Mars.

Different rovers had tried to find life in different places and had always found tantalising hints that life perhaps had been there but never any sign that life was there. It turns out they had been searching in the wrong places. Now this was going to start a whole new way of viewing Mars, a new set of explorations and new understandings. The man wrote up his notes, wrote up his personal log of what he had been up to for the day, he sent messages to his family back home to update them on his discovery and as the Martian day drew to a close, he went and had something to eat, spent a bit of time socialising and excitedly sharing his story, his discovery, how he has probably made history here on Mars, probably the first significant bit of true honest Martian history since people settled here. Then he went to bed for the night looking forward to waking up and continuing his study in the morning, continuing to see if other caves held life, continuing to find other caves and seeing if there are other locations this kind of life can survive in. And he drifted and fell comfortably, relaxed, asleep.

Lost City in the Woods

Steps for increasing effectiveness of the story:

1. What do you want to achieve from reading this?

2. Think about one thing you have achieved today.

3. Say to yourself "When I read this story then…"

Alternative introduction:

"As I read this and begin to drift comfortably asleep, I don't know whether I will find myself drifting asleep more to the sound of my voice or the words I read, or perhaps to the spaces between the words. And as I drift comfortably asleep I'll just read this story to myself."

So, as you listen to me, you can begin to drift comfortably asleep and while you begin to drift comfortably asleep you can allow yourself to get comfortable and allow your eyes to close. And I don't know whether you will drift off to sleep with the words that I use, with the sound of my voice, or perhaps with the spaces between my words.

And you can have a sense of being out bird watching one day. Of being in a little shed, a little bird watching shack, with some binoculars gazing out from this quiet spot. And you are gazing out through some woodland, over a large valley and you can see different birds in the nearby bits of woodland, but you can also see a large circling bird of prey in the distance in the valley and you can see it so gracefully circling. Seeming to use almost no effort and you look through binoculars at that graceful bird of prey and you have that unusual experience where, when you watch that through binoculars you shut off from the reality around you and awareness of the shack and awareness of everything else, to almost like you are very near to the bird, almost flying with them.

And while you watch that bird flying so gracefully and effortlessly, you begin to have a sense of thinking what it must be like to be able to fly like that, to be able to drift around in the sky, to rise up on warm air currents, circle round, to have the excellent vision of that bird. To see so clearly and so far and you can find yourself imagining that so strongly, that all of a sudden you become the bird. Seeing through the bird's eyes, flying drifting, soaring high in the sky, feeling weightless, floating, circling around, seeing woodland in the distance, seeing the vast expanse of the valley, green grass. Noticing bits of movement jump out at you as creatures scurry around on the ground. Seeing the way, the tops of the trees vibrate in the breeze and just feeling that sense of calmness, of peace and simplicity, at just flying and floating so gracefully with so little effort.

And while you continue to fly gracefully, you start exploring. And it is as if somehow you have taken over this bird. And a part of you is thinking 'Am I still in the shack watching the bird and somehow, I have drifted into a daydream, or was I watching the bird so intensely that I have got into the bird's psyche, somehow managed to get into the bird's mind?'. And either way, you go with the experience. You notice this fast-flowing river and you decide to soar down, fly over that water and you take some time to soar down and fly over the water, going in the direction the water is going, as it cascades down different waterfalls around rocks, through rapids and you fly just above the water, feeling the spray from the water, smelling the water, hearing the water, as it roars in rapids and then goes almost silent in calm areas. And you notice if you get just the right point above the water you can feel that you are flying on a cushion of air between the water and your wings. And so, you fly on that cushion of air and glide and float and follow that river all the way down to a lake. And as you reach the beginning of the lake you soar up into the air and circle around again and think of the fun you are having, as a bird flying, taking all of this in.

You feel a sense of elegance and grace and you continue exploring. And you are now in an area you have never been before. As a bird watcher you have been and watched birds before. You have even been down and walked through the valley, you have even walked and seen some of that river and the lake, but now you seem to have flown over an area you have never been before. An area of woodland, only you notice something about this woodland.

Your eyesight is so good that you notice subtleties, you notice that some trees are slightly higher up than others and you notice there is a certain pattern to these trees and intuitively something tells you it is worth going down there and investigating. So you fly down and you are too big to fit through the treetops in this area of the woodland, so you circle around and explore and conclude that you are going to have to land at the beginning of the woodland, but you don't know how well a bird of prey is going to be able to walk from the beginning of the woodland all the way into the woods, but you don't see an alternative, so you fly around and land at the beginning of the woodland and as you come in to land, you bring your wings back, you open them wide, slowing you right down, catching as much wind as possible, catching as much of that air as possible. And you put your feet out in front of you and you have an odd experience, that just as your feet touch the ground, you become yourself again and you find yourself stood before the woodland.

You are still trying to work out whether this is a dream and whether you have somehow gazed at that bird so intensely that you are now dreaming and having this experience and yet it feels very real and undream-like. And you think, if it was just a dream wouldn't you just wake up by just deciding this is a dream and deciding to just wake up and yet it doesn't seem like a dream or something you can wake up from. It's not something that bothers you, it is just a curiosity.

You walk into the woods, listening to the footsteps, listening to the different sounds in the woods, noticing how the light changes as you walk into the woods. And the woods are quite dense and you have to push through and work your way through. And as you push and work your way through the woods, you notice that there are some areas that seem to be a bit higher, areas that seem to be a bit lower, like the woods have built on top of something. But you don't know what and you keep pushing and pushing, until eventually there is an area that is a little bit clearer and you notice that the woods have overgrown over some kind of old building. And as you walk around and explore, you find that it seems to have grown over lots of old buildings.

You keep walking and keep exploring and all you keep finding is more and more buildings like this is a huge area of many buildings. Then you find a bit that looks like a normal bit of land, perhaps a normal outcrop of rock and you decide to go and explore it and you scratch through the plants that have covered it over and you notice that it is a wall of a building that has partially collapsed. And you follow this wall to see where it leads. It seems like you have found some kind of building that would have been near the centre of this lost city. Then as you keep exploring, you notice an indentation in the ground and you notice that this is where an entrance must have once been. So, you start clearing this entrance space and you find that just behind a bit of rubble is a tunnel heading downwards with some steps.

You walk in to the tunnel and as you do, somehow, oddly, your eyes adapt to be able to see in this tunnel, like somehow you have got some of the abilities of the wild animals in this area. You don't try to understand it because you are too busy thinking that it benefits what you want to achieve, you want to explore this area. So, you head down deeper into this building. And quite a way down you find a stone slab that you think is probably in front of an entrance to something. And you start pushing around on the stone slab and around on the wall around the stone slab and then somehow, you just take a step and the slab moves aside. And it grinds and moves aside, as you walk through and you find yourself in a vast chamber.

Within this vast chamber, you notice that there are scrolls all around the walls in diamond shaped spaces and there has got to be tens of thousands of scrolls in the spaces around the walls, perhaps like some lost civilisations' library. You manage to carefully open one of the scrolls and it is in a language you don't understand, so you put it back and you open another one and it is in the same language that you don't understand so you put it back and you suspect there is so much wisdom contained within these scrolls. And you see, right in the middle of the room is a pedestal with an open scroll and the scroll is being held open with a golden clasp at the top and the bottom and you stand in front of that scroll, you stand near the pedestal and you assume you aren't going to be able to read this one either and you gaze at this scroll and everything on it begins to change, almost like a mist passing across the scroll. And it is like the writing is rewriting itself and the scroll ends up being able to be read, it ends up readable and so you start reading this scroll and realise it is teaching you inner wisdom, it is teaching you something that will transform your life.

You read the scroll with fascination, with wonder, only vaguely aware of the impact it is going to have positively on you. And you read that this one also includes instructions saying that all the scrolls can be read when held on this pedestal by this golden clasp. So, you go and get another scroll, you place that on the pedestal and clasp it into place and you watch as the writing transforms, almost like mist and movement and changing of the text, to become readable. And you read that one and it is full of knowledge you never would have known, ancient knowledge, ancient wisdom. Then you get another scroll, putting that one back and notice that that scroll also contains ancient wisdom. And you wonder how long it would take to work your way through the thousands of scrolls full of ancient wisdom in this place. And you read another scroll and another scroll. Taking in and learning more ancient wisdom. Learning on an instinctive level. Learning that with a certain focus, you can become the animals, you can join the spirit of the animals and somehow you had stumbled across that focus and by stumbling across that focus, allowed you to stumble across this knowledge. And you read and learn and find this knowledge fascinating. And you realise it would take too long to learn all of this knowledge right now, you decide to continue exploring.

And so, you put the original scroll back in place on the pedestal and make sure all the other scrolls are put away in their places and you explore deeper and deeper into this space. And as you explore, so you discover a giant underground lake and on that lake is a boat and this lake is totally still and you feel it is so still that it is almost unnaturally still, but then, there is no breeze down here.

You get into the boat and row that boat to the other side of the lake and get out of the boat. And you can now see that the lake has ripples and you wonder how much those ripples will die down by the time you pass across that lake as you return. And you carry on exploring, wondering who created this whole underground space, where underneath this city there is a vast lake and why did they create it? And you see some statues and you see giant pearls and crystals in the walls and you notice how they appear to be glowing, as if maybe there was tubes of light coming in from above, lighting up the back of the pearls and crystals. And you find a chamber and on a shelf in that chamber is the most elegant item of clothing you have ever seen. So beautifully woven. Something handcrafted that you know would have taken years to make. And you know this shows the amount of skill these people had, even though you don't know who these people are.

Then you see a puzzle on the wall and you know there is no further to go in this chamber, but you think it is curious having a puzzle, so you try and solve the puzzle. And after a while moving things around, trying to work the puzzle out, suddenly you get the puzzle, something inside you clicks and makes it make sense to you and then a secret door opens. You go through the secret door, going deeper and deeper into this building. And you see a room so large that you can't see the other side of it. You can't see the side on the left or the side on the right, you don't know how the ceiling is being held up in a room this large. And you walk into the room and after a very, very long time of walking in a straight line so that you don't get lost, just following the markings on the ground, you find yourself at another pedestal, only on this pedestal is a bit confusing, you see a perfectly polished black pebble.

And so, you pick up that perfectly polished black pebble, you feel it in your fingers, you run it through your fingers, feel the smoothness of that pebble. You then see a note next to the pebble that says 'Take me.'.

And then you turn the note over and it says 'Put me in your shoe and lose me, when the time is right.".

And you think that this is unusual, but you take the pebble, you slide it into the side of your shoe, feeling it is a bit uncomfortable, but you slide it into the side of your shoe, you don't know why you followed these instructions but you feel these people must have a reason and you are curious what that reason may be and you know the only way to discover the reason is to follow along, so you put that pebble in your shoe. And you find your way, with a bit of a limp initially, out of that room and you start finding your way back through the building. After a while, you habituate to that pebble in your shoe and you stop noticing the pebble in your shoe and you know it is still there and you know that if you draw attention to it, you notice it again.

You continue to find your way out and then find your way into the woods. Then you work your way through the wood, back the way you came and when you exit the woods, you don't know how far it is to get back to where you came from. You know you are supposed to be birdwatching, but you don't know how to get back to where you are birdwatching. And then you feel this compulsion to jump. And you jump up in the air and instantly, you seem to have wings and you do a large flap and launch yourself higher into the air and you notice you are that bird again and you fly and you catch an updraft of warm air and you spiral round and rise up higher into the air. You don't give it any thought, you just seem to know your way back to where you were first seen as a bird and you fly your way back to that location and circle around in that location and the next minute you feel a slight curious feeling and realise you are looking through some binoculars at the bird and you wonder whether that was all a dream and are curious what it was all about. Then you look down and notice you have a pebble in your shoe and realise it wasn't all a dream. Something happened, some experience. And you don't know what it all means and you decide to follow those instructions of keeping that pebble in your shoe until such time as it is just naturally time to lose the pebble. And so that is what you decide to do.

Past-Life Regression

Steps for increasing effectiveness of the story:

1. What do you want to achieve from reading this?

2. Think about one thing you have achieved today.

3. Say to yourself "When I read this story then…"

Alternative introduction:

"As I read this and begin to drift comfortably asleep, I don't know whether I will find myself drifting asleep more to the sound of my voice or the words I read, or perhaps to the spaces between the words. And as I drift comfortably asleep I'll just read this story to myself."

This bedtime story is about someone visiting a hypnotist for past-life regression. And so, you will be taking on the role of that person visiting the hypnotist for past-life regression.

And as you listen to this, make sure it is at a time when you can relax fully, when you can pay this your full attention, when you won't be disturbed, when you can just drift, comfortably asleep. And as you listen to this and drift comfortably asleep I don't know whether you will fall asleep faster because of the words I use, because of the sound of my voice, or perhaps the spaces between my words. So, while you drift comfortably asleep, I'll guide you through this story.

So, you decide one day that you are curious about past-life regression, you are curious about whether you have lived before and if you have lived before, what did you do, who were you, what were your past lives like? So, you visit a hypnotist and when you turn up at the hypnotists' office, he guides you into his room where you see this incredibly comfy chair. He suggests you take a moment to sit comfortably in that chair, to make yourself comfortable in that chair. To take a few comfortable breaths. And to just let relaxation happen. And you don't necessarily know how to just let relaxation happen, so you just sit in the chair and you notice that the chair is so comfortable that your shoulders begin to relax, the chair is so comfortable that your back begins to relax, that your bottom and your legs begin to relax, that your arms and hands begin to relax. And you notice how all of this is happening, automatically and instinctively. You are not trying to make any of this happen, it is just happening automatically and instinctively. And as your body continues to relax, so your eyes get heavy and as they get heavier and heavier, you notice how the eyelids, blink, shut.

And as the eyelids shut all by themselves, so a wave of relaxation spreads down your body from the top of your head, all the way down to the tips of your toes. And the hypnotist hasn't even started talking yet. All of this has happened just because the chair was so comfortable, just so, incredibly comfortable. Then the hypnotist gently leans forward and says

"That's right, relaxing, deeper and deeper, becoming more and more relaxed, as you listen to the sound of my voice and as you listen to the sound of my voice, so you will begin to journey back in time. You will begin to journey back in time. To a time before you were born.".

And as the hypnotist talks to you and tells you these things, your mind begins to wander backwards in time. And you feel a certain warmth, or pressure, or heaviness, or a certain sensation, as you drift deeper into the experience. And as your mind drifts back in time and initially you just get flashes and glimmers of light and subtle elements of images. And then these elements of images and these flashes of light, start to form into something more.

And it is almost as if you just blink, once, or twice, or three times and open your eyes, finding yourself laying on a cobbled street, hearing some bells in the background, the clippity-clop of some horses and carts wheels on the cobbled street. The sounds of people chattering and getting on with daily life. As you feel the cobbles beneath your hands and your legs as you are laying there, wondering where you are, what this life is.

And as you look around yourself, you see a nearby pub and you feel a bit woozy and you realise you must have been drinking in the pub and perhaps you have fallen over when you came out. And you look around and you can smell the air. And you can sense the atmosphere and you feel warm and happy. And you gaze over and through a slight haze, you see people having fun, enjoying themselves.

And then you see a newspaper seller, a boy standing on a street corner and you go over and have a look at the paper and see the date, 1874. And you notice that the paper is a London paper. And you start exploring this past-life. Exploring London in 1874. And by this point, the hypnotist's voice seems to have just vanished into the background, as you become more and more absorbed in the past-life. And you look for what you can learn about yourself from this past-life. Why this life, what does it mean, what does it teach you? And you explore the life. And then as you become more deeply absorbed in the experience and you explore and you go to the River Thames and you have a look at the Thames and you see sail boats heading down the river and you notice what the sun looks like in the sky, what the clouds look like. And as you gaze at the sun and clouds, so things begin to change. And almost like a merging of images you find yourself standing in a university campus on a path, at a crossroads on that path.

And the path is quite white and the grass is very green and there are plenty of trees. And you notice from what the buildings look like and from the way people are dressed that this must be the 1700's. You ask someone as they walk nearby for the exact date. They say it is April 4th 1763. And you wonder what relevance or meaning this must have for you. Why did you end up here? And you explore this past-life. And it can seem so real. Seeing what you see, hearing what you hear, feeling what you feel. And every now and then, you just get a glimmer of the hypnotist's voice in the background, but mostly you are in this past-life that is like leading a real life. And you wonder what you are supposed to learn here. And you continue exploring this life and you realise that you have a ring with you and that you plan on proposing, but you don't know who to or why, or what the relationship is like, but you take some time to find out.

And then after a while, the university campus begins to change again and you have a sense of drifting back, deeper and deeper in time. And the university seems to be transforming into a pyramid. And the grass seems to be turning sandy. And you discover yourself in ancient Egypt. At a time when Gods were virtually real. When the pharaohs were thought to be the Gods and Gods were thought to come out at night and come out in the morning and to influence the world around them. And you are working hard, dragging a giant stone with 100 other people. You can notice the tension in the legs, dragging that stone. The effort that is required. Wondering what you are learning from this experience.

And you continue to explore the experience, unaware of how guided you are by the hypnotist, you barely notice the hypnotist's voice in the background, as you are absorbed in the past-life. After a short while, you get an epiphany and suddenly realise the connection between the lives, between the roles that you have been taking, you suddenly learn something about yourself. Some inner discovery, some inner wisdom. And once you discover this, you start making your journey back to the hypnotist's office through one past life, then the other, then the other. Working your way back to the hypnotist's office, where you find yourself deeply hypnotised.

And as the story comes to an end when you reach the office and when the hypnotist brings that you round, you can continue drifting deeper into a comfortable sleep, drifting off comfortably, deeply asleep. Soundly, comfortably, deeply, asleep. Finding it easy and effortless to drift.......off.......to.......sleep.

Past-Life Regression

Printed in Great Britain
by Amazon